OKLAHOMA CITY, APRIL 1995

The crowds got bigger as the team got closer to the Myriad Center. They lined the pavement as if drawn by some invisible force, yet the quiet remained unbroken. Faces along the route were wet with tears that no one tried to hide.

Then Beth heard a voice cut the still morning as in prayer. "Yea, though I walk through the valley of the shadow of death, I shall fear no evil." It was a final, wrenching homage to the victims of the bombing. The voice echoed inside Beth's head. "I shall fear no evil," she chanted over and over again, trying desperately to keep her feelings at bay.

Beth felt her anger melt away. She and Czar would be all right; she'd make sure of that. The people of Oklahoma had reminded them of what their volunteer of love was all about. The motto of search and rescue—to save lives and reduce human suffering—made it all worthwhile for her and the white shepherd.

SEARCH AND RESCUE

Samantha Glen and Mary Pesaresi

FAWCETT CREST • NEW YORK

A Fawcett Crest Book
Published by Ballantine Books
Copyright © 1997 by Samantha Glen and Mary Pesaresi

All rights reserved under International and Pan-American Copyright Conventions. Published in the United States by Ballantine Books, a division of Random House, Inc., New York, and simultaneously in Canada by Random House of Canada Limited, Toronto.

http://www.randomhouse.com

Library of Congress Catalog Card Number: 96-90774

ISBN 0-449-22578-X

Manufactured in the United States of America

First Edition: April 1997

10 9 8 7 6 5 4 3 2 1

This book is dedicated with admiration and respect to all the wonderful men, women, and dogs of Search and Rescue.

To save lives and
reduce human suffering
SEARCH AND RESCUE MOTTO

ACKNOWLEDGMENTS

This book was a labor of love. The endless hours, boundless patience, and dedication to search and rescue that is the common thread binding the men and women and dogs to their task is likewise a labor of love. This was one among many things Beth Barkley taught us about the volunteer vocation to which she has committed her life.

We wish to thank Heidi Yamaguchi of DOGS East, Penny Sullivan of the American Rescue Dog Association, and Hatch and Judy Graham of the California Rescue Dog Association for sharing their knowledge; Bev and Larry Peabody and Shirley Hammond of CARDA, and Captain Garrett Dwyer of FEMA's Virginia Task Force #1 for further insights into the workings of SAR; and the personnel of FEMA (Office of Federal Emergency Management Agency) and members of police, fire, and medical teams nationwide who also contributed to the overall mosaic of SAR.

But especial thanks must go to the following four people: Andy Rebmann and Marcia Koenig, owners of one of the best training schools for SAR dogs in America, K-9 Speciality Search School of Redmond, Washington; Skip Fernandez of the Special Operations Division, Metro-Dade Fire Department; and Kevin George of the Search and Rescue Dog Association of Alberta, Canada. The endless hours graciously spent by these men and women to help us "get it right" was above and beyond the call of duty and sincerely appreciated.

And this book could not have come into being without our editor, Elisa Wares, who loved the project from its inception; our agent, Meredith Bernstein, who labored alongside us, always in our corner; and Elizabeth Cavanaugh, her right hand, who delved enthusiastically into the undertaking and kept the faith.

Our sincere thanks to one and all.

AUTHORS' NOTE

Search and Rescue is a book of one woman's recollections of her years in volunteer search and rescue work. Dialogue must necessarily be reconstructed, but this and all events are depicted as accurately as memory and reconstruction will allow.

THE MARCH OF SILENCE

Oklahoma City, Sunday, April 30, 1995, 8:00 A.M.

The dog sat, his massive head hanging in weariness. The German shepherd could barely wag his tail as his mistress attempted to pat the fine glaze of cement dust from his stiff white fur. Day after day of death had taken its toll on Czar.

The woman knelt beside him, drawing her brush in deliberate strokes along the length of his body. The dog leaned against her as if to take comfort from the familiar ritual. An overwhelming anger threatened to shatter the outward calm the woman had so carefully cultivated the past week. The long nights of searching for bodies in the crumpled remains of the Alfred P. Murrah Federal Building seemed to have broken her partner's spirit—and very nearly her own.

This was not the Czar she knew—the animal who would jump up and nearly spit in her face with excitement when he'd made a "find," the rambunctious canine who'd yatter, yatter, yatter like a woodpecker on a tree when he wanted her to follow closely. This was a Czar steeped in exhaustion.

She was glad the team was being sent home tomorrow. Eight days they'd been there, joining other search-and-rescue crews from California, Arizona, New York, Maryland, and Florida. Eight nights of freezing twelve-hour shifts, sifting through rubble to recover yet another body part. The woman understood better than most how important it was to return people's remains to their families. Human beings the world over seemed to need to see the body to fully understand that a loved one was dead; seemed to need the closure of burial. It is the first step toward grieving and eventual healing.

But now there was nothing more the Task Force from Fairfax, Virginia could do here—nothing more anyone could do. The woman stroked the back of the dog beside her. "Not long now, boy."

Beth Barkley eased her tired body upward and rolled her head from side to side. The little clicks of release that sounded in her neck made her feel better. She glanced around the garage that had been the staging area for the sixty-two men and women who had come with her to Oklahoma. The cavernous space was unnaturally still on this, their last morning. Task Force #1 got ready in quiet seriousness for what they were about to do.

Some wiped at the dust that clung to their faces like gray snow. Others smacked the dirt from their navy coverups. Some shared combs. The other three dog handlers brushed and watered their animals, just as she tended the creamy white shepherd who hid his face against her belly.

Beth recognized the detached withdrawal she saw around her. It was a discipline of the work, this self-imposed numbness, required of dog and human alike. Emotion was dangerous when recovering the shattered remnants of once living beings, when moving tons of rubble by hand in yellow, five-gallon buckets. The focus must be on the search. There was no time to react to the sights, smells, and sounds of those moments. But now, at the end of this mission, Beth had a few minutes to think—dangerous.

Like a silent movie the images played on the screen of her mind: Czar's drooping head as he pawed at the giant slab of stone that would expose the remains of a black marine, dusted with debris except for his spit-shined shoes; Czar's ears pressed back against his head as the team formed a corridor of sympathy for the Oklahoma City firefighter whose sister had been lifted from the rubble. Czar's body language reflected everyone's quelled emotions.

Beth tried to reason her feelings. She was a veteran of other devastations: earthquakes in El Salvador and Armenia, floods in West Virginia, mud slides in Virginia, and more. She'd spent many hours pondering those capricious events called "disasters." Hurricanes, earthquakes, and tornadoes had always seemed part of the natural order of things to her. Never had she felt any anger toward the events themselves.

But it had never been like this. Never before had the tragedy come at the hands of man. The anger welled up more strongly than before.

"Let's go, guys." It was Garrett Dyer, their search team leader.

Beth was grateful it was about to begin. She buried her face in the ruff of the patient animal beside her. "Okay, boy," she whispered, "this is for them."

They lined up four abreast, Garrett insisting the dogs be in front. One last flick of the patches that told the world they'd come from Fairfax, Virginia—one quick blur of heads held high, shoulders straightened—and in squadron formation the men, women, and dogs who'd come to Oklahoma City marched out to the street.

The day was crisp and clear, sun-washed of the bitter, gray overcast that had chilled the air and soul since April 19. There was no commuter traffic, but people were out and about. The early strollers stopped and stared as the rescue workers walked the double-yellow ribbon dividing the avenue that led to the Myriad Center. Then the spectators clapped and cheered.

"Thank you so much," someone called.

"We love you," shouted another.

"God bless you," came another voice.

There was no response from the sixty-two people marching the line. They couldn't wave, couldn't return the smiles.

Silence descended on the crowd, its noise muted by waves of emotion. The hands came down, the smiles faded. And suddenly it was as if everyone understood.

This silent march was a tribute. One unit's response to the violation of the ordinary people who, one spring morning, had gotten out of bed, saw their children off to school, fed their animals, and reported to work. One team's expression of outrage at the monstrous crime committed against those who'd come to the credit union hoping they could afford a car, or to the Housing and Urban Development office to see about a place to live, or to the Social Security office to ask questions about their retirement years. One force's deep, deep sorrow for the children left for a few hours in day care, waiting trustfully for evening time when mommy or daddy would come to get them.

The crowds got bigger as the team got closer to the Myriad Center. They lined the pavement as if drawn by some invisible force, yet the quiet remained unbroken. Faces along the route were wet with tears that no one tried to hide.

Then Beth heard a voice cut the still morning as in prayer. "Yea, though I walk through the valley of the shadow of death, I shall fear no evil." It was a final, wrenching homage to the victims of the bombing. The voice echoed inside her head. "I shall fear no evil," she chanted over and over, trying desperately to keep her feelings at bay.

At last, the team reached the loading dock of the Myriad Center that had served as cafeteria, sleeping quarters, and gathering place for their time in Oklahoma City. They walked in straight as soldiers.

The area was crowded with the citizens who had fed and clothed them, put mints and dog treats on their pillows, tacked schoolchildren's notes of thanks and poems of encouragement to the walls. They, too, watched in silence as the team marched in.

Suddenly the place erupted with applause and cheers. And Task Force #1 from Fairfax, Virginia finally bowed to the emotions they'd held inside for so long.

They wept. They hugged. They said their thank-yous in return for all the deep, caring gratitude that washed over them.

Beth felt her anger melt away. She gazed fondly at her big dog, now surrounded by volunteers. She and Czar would be all right; she'd make sure of that. And together the partners would answer the next call. The people of Oklahoma had reminded them of what their volunteer of love was all about. The motto of search and rescue—to save lives and reduce human suffering—made it all worthwhile for her and the white shepherd.

It had been quite a journey for Czar and Beth, one that was far from over. A flash of memory from years past came to her: another shepherd; white, eyes of deepest brown, with manners befitting a duchess. Panda.

And in that moment, in that place, Beth Barkley wondered what road she might have traveled if it hadn't been for the other white dog.

It all began with Panda.

PART ONE

EARLY DAYS

CHAPTER 1

PANDA

Falls Church, Virginia, August 11, 1980

The blue Mustang lurched to a stop in its normal parking spot outside Beth Barkley's little house. She opened the door, but made no move to exit the car; she just sat, feeling the sweat bead on her brow. What was her problem?

Doc had been gone for months now, yet she couldn't seem to stop mourning her beloved Dalmatian. Maybe it wasn't just Doc's death. Beth was only thirty-six and in the best of health, but maybe the 100-degree heat and humidity that had steamed the East Coast all month added to her irritability; maybe the unusually heavy load at work caused this feeling of general malaise.

The slim, lovely woman with smoke-green eyes lifted the heavy strands of waist-length blond hair from her neck and hoped for a cooling breeze that wasn't to be found. Her front door stared at her, called to her. She had to go in sometime. She walked to the door, and turned the knob.

"Surprise!"

The sound almost made her scream and run. A roomful of people smiled, waved, laughed, and elbowed one another with the success of their scheme.

"Oh, boy," she muttered just as someone thrust a glass of tepid champagne into her hand.

A handsome, second-generation Puerto Rican man, whose light coloring betrayed his English heritage, stepped forward and gathered her in his arms. "Happy marriage, darling," her new husband Jed murmured.

"Same to you," Beth answered.

"I've something special for you," Jed pronounced, leading her into the room.

"What?"

"Look around," he answered.

"You can't miss it," someone yelled, and everybody giggled.

Some joke at my expense, no doubt, Beth thought, still smiling, feeling her cheeks beginning to quiver with the effort.

It took a few seconds before she spotted the white German shepherd puppy trapped among her laughing friends.

Beth watched the animal shy away from first one person then another as it emitted pathetic whines. "What's that dog doing here, Jed?"

"Ah," her husband said, taking her hand and pulling her toward the pup. "Her name is Panda. She's a special wedding gift to you."

The strained smile was gone now. Beth lifted her gaze from the poor animal and looked daggers at her husband. "How could you do this so soon after Doc's death? I can't keep it. I'm *not* keeping it."

"She'll be fine once she gets used to us."

"I don't need this, Jed."

The white dog sniffed in their direction, then padded over. Pleading eyes fastened on Beth's. They were the color of fine porcelain painted deepest brown. Depending on the light, they could look chocolate, or darken to black. China-dish eyes. The shepherd was huge for a yearling, but her expression was appealing, and Beth smiled in spite of herself. The dog nudged closer. Beth's fingers edged out to meet rough, snowy fur. Panda sighed, and leaned the full weight of her body against the woman.

"I can take her to the shelter if you want," Jed offered.

A hard, bony head nuzzled under her hand. "In the morning," Beth answered.

For months Beth wondered why she'd said such a thing. Panda carried herself like a queen, although occasionally proving that even royalty has its bad moments. Every time the dog was left alone, she would destroy something. One day, Panda ate the kitchen cabinets a splinter at a time. Another day, Jed's beloved aquarium lay smashed in a million shards on the hardwood floor; Beth's house plants had been used as weapons to smear the doomed fish into her hooked rug.

This was not all Beth had to contend with. She had drifted away from her career as a classical singer, no longer performing with Leonard Bernstein, and world-class orchestras like the Royal Philharmonic, and she'd given up her teaching career, too.

Beth, who loved the outdoors, had grown tired of being cooped up inside with an office job. Her life seemed a tunnel with no end, no escape, and no variations.

Six months after the fateful wedding celebration, Beth came home, scooped up the *Fairfax Journal* from the lawn, absently fed the dog, and plopped down at the kitchen table, too weary to inspect the house for Panda's latest faux pas. Maybe this time Beth's mattress had been chewed up, or her books had been attacked. This kind of unpleasant little surprise could wait. She didn't have the energy to contend with it just now.

A headline in the paper caught Beth's eye, and she read on.

HERO DOGS

The hardworking animals of DOGS East have been saving lives, helping the police find evidence, and rescuing lost souls in the wilderness for about five years.

This is a volunteer organization, one of a few to be found across the country. The members are not compensated, and all expenses for dog and handler alike come out of their individual pockets, or from sporadic donations from individuals or organizations.

The work is not for everyone.

"It takes a certain type of dog," one of the handlers stated. "A dog that has great play drive, is highly intelligent, and has energy to spare. We're always looking for volunteers."

The more Beth read, the more intrigued she was. She glanced at Panda, and saw the animal's eager, intelligent eyes filled with life and energy.

"I think I've discovered something that's going to be good for both of us, Pan." She sighed, reaching for a scissors to clip out the article. "At least let's give it a try."

As if in answer, Pan put her head on Beth's lap and snorted contentedly.

"That sounds like a big 'yes' to me." Beth laughed.

CHAPTER 2

QUEEN OF THE PACK

October 1982, Prince William County, Virginia

The crunch of leaves underfoot and the steady ping of rain were the only sounds in the forest. Panda loped ahead—belly low to the ground, nose scenting a string-thin path through the decayed vines and creepers.

Beth lifted her collar against the wet, and hugged her body for warmth as she slouched after her dog. At least Pan didn't seem affected by the weather. Her thick, double coat protected her from the autumn storm as she worked her search pattern.

After two years, Beth knew her dog. She had become accustomed to the large, yet fine-boned body, and had learned to read the expressive eyes. She rather liked that Panda didn't have the ugly doggedness of a bloodhound, or the "hiya, hiya, hiya" friendliness of a golden retriever. Panda was elegant.

How many times had Beth watched the white shepherd sit in tranquil silence in the midst of turmoil—so still, so compelling, even the most dog-shy person would reach out a hand. Pan would respond by inching forward until the narrow of her neck was caressed by outstretched fingers.

Panda was tall, and she was gentle to the beings she considered her pack. No one had to bend to pet this dog.

Just now she roamed back and forth, in and out of a narrowing cone of scent that spiraled on the breeze from a human victim lost somewhere ahead. Pan rode the wind to the rescue.

Beth studied the grid pattern of her topographical map. Their quarter square mile of forest was marked by natural barriers: an ancient railroad track on the north, a stream festooned with leaves on the south. She checked her compass to make sure they were on track.

Suddenly, Panda froze and a high whine rumbled from her throat. The dog's alert was insistent. Beth sniffed hard in response, but her puny nose only pulled in the musk of rotting leaves, not the perfume Panda could smell so clearly—human.

"*¿Dónde está?*" Beth's question was quick and in Spanish, the language of choice in their home before she and Jed had split up a few months before.

Panda's thick fringe of tail painted a slow flag-wave left to right. One blurring movement, and the dog breached the barrier of branch and bush—then disappeared. A minute later she bounded back into sight through the dense thicket, eyes wide, ears pointed in excitement. One snort at her mistress and she was wheeling back the way she'd come. "*Si!*" Beth shouted, crashing in her wake. "Yes!" Panda was leading them toward her discovery in a perfect "recall/refind."

The body lay curled in a fetal position, hidden under a handful of dried ferns. "*Bueno, perrita de mi corazón,*" Beth praised as Pan pranced around her "find." She flicked open her radio. "Base camp, this is Beth. We found him. Over."

A broken crackle of noise jarred the quiet. "Good job."

Beth dropped to her knees beside the "victim," but he was already sitting up, shaking leaves from his parka. "Thank God, she only took thirty-five minutes," he said. "I don't mind volunteering to play 'missing' when it's sunny and seventy, but today . . ." The man who'd played dead jumped to his feet and grinned his appreciation at his "rescuers."

"Here, girl." He thumped Panda on her flanks, and produced a well-chewed Frisbee from behind his back. Panda's fangs clamped down hard. The man held on to one end of the toy while she growled and worried the other side. Back and forth, back and forth they tussled until the dog finally pulled the toy free. Pan leaped away—satisfied with a full measure of play as her reward for a job well done.

"By the way, what did you say to her just now?" he asked.

"*Perrita de mi corazón?* It's Spanish for 'little girl dog of my heart.' "

"That's beautiful."

It was a moment of triumph for Beth and her *perrita*—they had passed the last of the tests to qualify them as a search-and-rescue team. It had taken two years. Two years of training twice a week after work and most weekends. Two years of scrambling through woods, crawling under buildings, sloshing through swamp and stream.

Nothing had come easy. Right away, Beth was "volunteered" to play the "victim," hidden all over Virginia. Then it was her turn to train Panda—through swamps, across farms, up mountains. The team prepared for the worst that nature and man could devise.

In the first months, Panda was being bullied by Buster, a Rottweiler, and Kerry, a German shepherd. Not a training session passed without the dogs snapping at her rear. Finally, Panda's regal restraint deserted her. One frosty morning, she turned and nipped the snouts of her tormentors until they ran. Panda was now queen of DOGS East, and Beth's wallet was open to every vet in Virginia.

But the white shepherd was amazing. Her sensitive olfactory organs could detect and differentiate tiny fragments of scent hundreds of yards away, buried under mountains of rubble, or covered by fathoms of water. Her 220 million scent receptors overpowered Beth's mere human 20 million. Panda's finely honed ears could pinpoint the slightest sound; her intelligent eyes could focus on details her mistress needed binoculars to see. The woman stood in awe of her animal.

Panda wasn't the only one learning. Beth had to grasp how to set up a field command system, decipher topographical maps, and study wind currents and weather systems. She had to learn the variety of patterns a lost person might follow; it made a difference whether a victim was a hunter, a senior citizen, or a child.

The new team had to undergo obedience training, as well as agility tests that had them climbing ladders, jumping from trucks, crawling through culvert pipes, balancing on precarious platforms, pawing through rubble piles, and huddling in the bucket of front-end loaders high over the ground.

Beth and Panda loved every minute of it, and becoming a SAR team filled Beth's life since she and Jed parted.

And now, on this rain-drenched October day in 1982,

two years after reading that fateful article in the *Fairfax Journal*, the two companions had reached their long-sought and much-worked-for goal. They were a certified team for DOGS East.

Voices hailed them when they emerged from the woods, volunteer victim in tow.

"Congratulations!"

"Good job."

"You're ready for the real thing now!"

Neither Beth nor Panda imagined how hard the real thing would be.

CHAPTER 3

WHAT ARE WE DOING HERE?

One Week Later

"Okay, girl, this is it. Our first official search." Beth had fallen into the habit of talking to Panda as the dog rode shotgun beside her. "Two Boy Scouts lost in Quantico, and we're going to help find them." The dog's ears pricked at the familiar command of "find 'em." She thrust her pink nose upward, almost hitting the roof of the car.

"You're ready." Beth laughed, and wished she had her dog's confidence. She swung the white Camaro Berlinetta onto the road leading to the marine base. Thousands of acres of fields and woods spread beside her. Years ago, Quantico was a farming community. The government had taken down the houses and barns, but in the spring you could still see the little family cemeteries marked with daffodils and crocuses. Nice place. So why was her mouth so dry, and her stomach so queasy?

Pan seemed to sense they were close. The dog began to groom herself into ever more queenly splendor. At the same time, Beth saw the crowd. They spilled over the crossroads up ahead like a herd of wildebeests. There were maybe 300, and all in camouflage—marines.

Beth let Panda out of the car and scanned the mass of people for canines, hoping to see her DOGS East buddies. A woman sporting a sergeant's three stripes detached herself from the throng and hurried toward her. "Are you DOGS East?"

"Yes, where are—?"

"Thank God! Tell us what to do. We're ready."

Beth froze, her mouth agape. "I . . . I . . . I . . ." *Aie, aie, aie, aie, aie!* "Me?"

The sergeant nodded—mercifully oblivious to Beth's dismay. "At your command, ma'am."

Marines. At her *command.* A wicked little notion stole into her mind. *Line 'em up from cute to ugly.* Beth smiled at the thought.

Two frown lines appeared between eyebrows in desperate need of plucking. "Ma'am?" the sergeant questioned.

Beth was finding it hard not to stare over the woman's shoulder. If she could see just one member of her group. *Rich? Bob? Marion? Anybody? Where are you?*

"Ma'am?" The sergeant's voice rose a notch, and her eyes narrowed.

"Do you have topographical maps of the area that show all roads—paved, gravel, farm lanes, hunters' trails?" Beth asked.

"Have 'em, ma'am," the sergeant replied.

"Good. Do you have pictures of the boys?"

"Yep. Copies made, too."

"Good work."

Panda yawned and looked toward the woods. When her mistress didn't budge, the dog sat, her nether regions hitting the road with a plop.

"Sorry, girl," Beth whispered. Her voice took on a

brisk authority. "Mark where those scouts disappeared. I'll check on wind direction and velocity for the dogs. Divide your people into groups of ten. When you're done, let me know. I'll have sectors on maps and hand out assignments."

Panda nudged Beth with her big muzzle, then turned her back on her mistress. The little griping sounds she'd been making for the last few minutes got louder by the second. Beth gave her a perfunctory pat. "I know, girl. I want to search, too."

Beth used the hood of the Camaro to lay out the maps. She'd been vaguely aware of a man in jeans and a parka standing nearby during her conversation with the sergeant. He approached now, and held out his hand. Beth absently shook it, but he didn't let her go. "One of those scouts is my boy. Can you find him?"

She looked up to see the man crying. His pain was palpable, and her sudden coldness had nothing to do with the chill of the night air. Life or death could depend on the orders *she* was about to give. "I'll do my best. Count on it."

One hour later, three hundred marines had fanned across the countryside. Beth took a minute to steady herself. It was too dark for the sergeant to see her pallor, and none of the soldiers could hear the pounding in her chest. The thought gave her a little relief. Maybe she'd carried it off with no one the wiser as to her inexperience.

A car skidded to a halt next to hers, carrying Marion Hardy and Rich Fifer from DOGS East, with their animals in tow. Beth could barely stop herself from kissing their boots.

"Marion!" she cried, happy her voice sounded normal.

"Beth!" Marion answered. "We thought you'd be here

first, since you're the closest. Show us what you've done."

There was never time for small talk when lives were in danger, and Marion and Rich were all business. They listened in silence as Beth explained the maps, how she had arranged the grids, and where she had deployed the volunteer searchers.

"Good job," Rich stated.

The ache of tension in Beth's neck eased. Thank God, she hadn't made any fatal blunders. "May I go search now?"

Her two companions from DOGS East grinned, and Beth had an uncomfortable realization that her fears weren't as well hidden as she had thought.

"Which section have you assigned yourself?" Rich asked.

Beth pointed to a small square on the map.

"Okay. Good luck."

Panda figured she'd waited long enough. She twisted around, nosing her orange shabrack, the jacket that was her search-dog uniform. She placed her front paws on the fender of the Camaro, her grumbling louder in the quieting night. "Okay. *Activa.*" Panda let out a joyful yip. Her mistress grabbed her hard hat and radio, and they headed for the woods.

Beth relished the crystalline night, more comfortable in her partnership with Panda than giving orders to the military. Within two hours, they were able to radio in an "all clear"—no scouts in her sector. That was something at least. Now if only the voice of some marine would echo over her radio with a "Found 'em."

She and Panda returned to base as fast as they could. Small knots of marines and a smiling Rich Fifer were waiting. "We just got the news. Two privates in a jeep located the scouts," Rich yelled. A cheer rose up around her. Beth laughed with them, but she was a little disappointed. She'd secretly hoped she and Panda would locate the boys.

"Hey, lady!" The dad of one of the scouts ran toward her. "Thanks. I never saw anything organized so fast in my life. You saved my boy."

Beth stared at the happy faces of those surrounding her. Rich was on the radio, broadcasting the good news to the other men and women who'd come to search. "It was all of us," Beth answered. "We're a team."

She stooped in front of Panda, and rubbed her. "Wow, this feels good," she whispered to her partner. "Want to do this again? Yeah, me, too."

Beth had only one regret as she drove away from the milling, celebrating bunch. She *should* have ordered those marines to line up from cute to ugly.

CHAPTER 4

LEARNING CURVE

"Local authorities call the Virginia Department of Emergency Services (VDES)." Beth's voice was sleep slurred. In fact, she *was* asleep—with a 600-page book clutched to her chest. "State police to local authorities to Virginia Department of Emergency Services. VDES." She'd dreamed the order of authority for search and rescue until she wanted to swat at it like a buzzing insect.

Beth rolled over and nearly fell on the floor. She grabbed her bedside table just in time. Panda had nudged her to the far edge again. How was it that the shepherd snored in all her royal glory, sprawled over three-quarters of the bed, while she, Beth, with the red eyes, was up studying at 2:00 A.M.? She pushed the white bulk of canine across the sheets, and restaked her claim to a skinny section of the mattress.

She closed her eyes and willed sleep. It was no use. "If you want to be a part of search and rescue, your group must have a Memorandum of Understanding with VDES. MOU. Memorandum of Understanding. MOU." Her inner voice droned on. "You must test to our standards. Must abide by our regulations. Must. Must . . ."

What exactly those regulations were, Beth hadn't yet gotten around to knowing. But after the search for the scouts in Quantico, she realized that trekking to seminars all over the country at no little expense, and being the mistress of the newest search dog on the East Coast, didn't change the fact that she was a rank novice when it came to search management—or MSO, "Managing the Search Organization," as it was officially titled at what amounted to the place for higher education in search and rescue—"SAR College."

And Beth wouldn't stand for that. She wanted to know this work inside and out—to become a coveted "state resource." It wasn't just a flattering title; it meant wearing her own beeper, so that she and Panda would be on direct call to the VDES at all times. She wanted to earn the distinction even if it killed her.

She squeezed her cramped shoulder blades. God, her back hurt. She used to think "if it killed her" was a flippant phrase. That was before she called Virginia Department of Emergency Services in an effort to continue her education in search work.

Within a week the textbooks arrived. And arrived. And arrived. Beth's head was getting crazy with it all. It didn't help that Panda snoozed in bed or under the cooling canopy of her favorite oak while Beth sweated the tomes.

More than once the woman wished she could change places with the dog. A hundred times she wondered how many search and rescue aspirants got this far and decided that this sort of volunteer work was not for them after all.

Then came notice of the classes: two forty-hour weekends, held at the 4-H Club facility near Front Royal, Virginia. Beth would have to bunk down in a four-person dorm. That was the easy part; from what she'd been told the accommodations were very comfortable, and the local ladies cooked up succulent meals for the students.

The sessions would start on a Friday evening (after the volunteers got off from their regular jobs) and continue through Sunday at 1700 hours. That's five in the afternoon, Beth thought, still having to make a conscious translation from military time.

And Beth would then know what it took to be an FTL—a Field Team Leader.

FTL, VDES, MOU, MSO. She swore it was remembering the words behind the abbreviations, not the actual training itself, that would trip her up.

During the second weekend they would put all their newly gained knowledge to work on a mock search. It would begin Saturday night before supper for some, after for others, and last well into the wee hours of Sunday morning.

Then, hallelujah, the next step. If the rigors of training didn't break her, and if she passed all the tests thrown at her by Ralph Wilfong, VDES search-and-rescue coordinator, she might be called upon to be an instructor herself. That might, just might, enhance her role as a state resource.

How many years down the line was that dream?

Panda turned and plopped her legs on Beth's tummy. The woman didn't have the energy to heave them off. She tried to remember the ease of her life before the white monster had pushed a bony head into her hand: the endless hours of leisure she'd had to go to the movies, visit friends, take a vacation. But something else had become more important.

The pure, unadulterated love that shone from Panda's eyes; the way that nobody bothered her when Pan would

park her square table of a body close to hers. The pleasure of seeing the dog run back on a search to make sure
she was okay. Her growing confidence that the dog
would never let her down. All these things comforted an
inner core of Beth's being that had never been touched
before. She sighed and switched on the light. "The duties
of the base commander are . . ."

They had so much to learn, she and Panda, and Beth
knew that the calls for them to respond to search-and-
rescue missions would continue unabated while they
studied and trained. But now it had become more than
simply a curiosity, more than an interest of Beth's. The
word "they" was correct; she was no longer in this alone.
It was understood now that Beth Barkley would go
nowhere without her partner.

CHAPTER 5

THE BUBBAS AND
THE BEAR

September 1984

It was one of those glorious fall mornings when the air was crisp and cool against the face, the sky brilliant and unclouded. The kind of morning fashioned by the gods for a dog and her mistress who had come to love the wilds of Virginia.

At least it would have been, but for the five "good ol' boys" snorting behind them. "Hold up, lady. What's your hurry?"

The complaint slowed Beth in midstride. She made no attempt to hide her annoyance. *"Aquí,"* she ordered, and the shepherd returned to her side.

Nothing had gone right today. Bob, the dispatcher, had called for her help in finding a missing hunter. After a five-hour drive into the mountains of the next state, to a place he'd described as "nearly nowhere," she was greeted by a sheriff's deputy she didn't know; and none of her DOGS East colleagues in sight. It didn't help that the "boys" the deputy had lined up as her guides seemed to think Panda was some kind of freak.

"She one of them albinos or something?" one of the hunters asked, pointing at Panda.

"No, her eyes are brown, not pink," Beth answered.

"Heard tell a good breeder kills them white ones when they come out."

"You 'heard tell' wrong," Beth was quick to reply. "Some breed *only* white-coated shepherds."

Where had the sheriff found these men? Not one of them weighed less than 250 pounds; all were larded with the muscle tone of mashed potatoes. These "boys," in their hunting orange with shotguns slung over their shoulders, were here to make sure *she* didn't get lost? She might end up having to save *their* lives.

"I don't need an escort," she said to the deputy. "I have a compass, map, and radio. My dog and I have been working a search every month for over two years."

The deputy's belly was only a few millimeters less in girth than those of her would-be guides. He hoisted the soft flesh a little higher and nodded toward the tapestry of rust and crimson that framed the wilderness. "No offense, ma'am, and we sure appreciate your coming, but I don't believe you or your dog know this area."

So Beth was stuck with the bubbas. "These gentlemen need to leave their guns here. They make the dog nervous. And I don't want any happy hunter mistaking Panda for a bear."

Her irony was completely lost on her companions. "We ain't got no polar bars here, lady."

"If you bring guns, I won't take one step with you."

"She's kiddin', right?" a hunter asked the deputy.

The deputy studied Beth's face for a moment and settled his hat way back on his head. "I think she means it, boys. Best leave your guns."

The "boys" headed reluctantly toward their trucks, muttering to each other. "We're ready," one of her escorts announced after all guns had been lovingly stowed in various pickups.

"I don't think quite yet." Beth eyed their tummies, which well deserved the name "beer guts." "We only take water to drink on a search."

"Water? You gotta be kidding, lady."

"Do what she says," the deputy snapped.

Packs were flung to the ground. Ten-inch zippers opened in unison. Thirty cans of beer, cosseted in padded coolers, got hauled into the sunlight. One guide handed his six-pack to the officer. "Keep 'em cold for us, will you, Deputy?"

"Sure, boys. No problem."

"Much appreciated, guys," Beth said and finally let Panda lead them into the forest.

Hours later, her scouts grumbling and whining every mile, Beth detected a change in the afternoon. The wind died, a drizzle began, and wisps of fog collected in the hollows. The temperature warmed for a while, then dropped ten degrees in fifteen minutes.

Panda bumped her from behind and trotted purposefully back the way they had come. "Pan, no. Get to work," Beth called. The shepherd came back reluctantly, circled her mistress, nudged her from behind again, and retreated.

Beth sniffed the air. What was that smell? "Pan, come back here," she called again. She felt an urgency, and turned to exhort her companions to move faster.

They were frozen behind her—transfixed as if turned into pillars of salt—staring slack-jawed into space. Suddenly, one came to life. "Bahr!" he yelled, and, like a herd of clumsy rhinos, the whole band took off.

"Bar?" Beth repeated to herself. Were they so desperate

for their lost six-packs they'd hallucinated some beer-joint? An abrupt powerful gust carried a strong scent to her. Panda, moving slowly toward her mistress, stiffened, and the almond ridge of fur rose along the shepherd's back. With sudden understanding, Beth knew what "bar" meant—*bear*.

The animal was upwind of them. It couldn't know they were there, or it would have been on them. Mercy! Her dog wouldn't stand a chance against the clawed beast.

Beth lurched forward. She clamped her hand around Panda's snowy muzzle and headed downwind as fast as the awkward arrangement would allow.

Cover. They needed cover. She skirted a clump of dying ferns that hugged a story-high outcropping of rock, let go Panda's muzzle and grabbed her ruff, forcing the shepherd's haunches to the ground beside her.

Beth inhaled long, slow breaths to calm herself. She peered around their refuge, back the way they'd come. Still she couldn't see the bear.

Then, suddenly, the animal came into view, and all Beth could think was how beautiful it was. The bear's coat was like sable velvet lit by candlelight, stirring in the wind as if ruffled by invisible fingers. The eyes were Panda's dark, burnished brown as they blinked against the thin shafts of sun. The animal scented exactly like Panda—nose high and proud, head swinging side to side, now and then brushing the tips of dying foliage. The bear was retracing the dog's steps.

Panda was coiled tension. She broke cover and stood guard—the age-old instinct to protect her mistress over-riding any command Beth could give. The woman was helpless as she watched the bear ease closer, scenting the path they'd taken.

It was a young bear, light on its feet, lacking the heaviness of maturity. The bear stopped, raised on its hindquarters. Had it seen Panda? Would the contrast of the dog's orange shabrack against white fur attract attention? Just how good or bad was a bear's eyesight? The dog made no move. Nor did the bear. Beth prayed wordlessly, fervently.

In a slow, liquid descent, Panda sat. From her throat curled a low rumble that Beth felt rather than heard. The bear's snout jabbed the air in the shepherd's direction; then it coughed, lowered slowly to the ground, and turned away. The last the woman saw was a smear of supple brown haunches melting into the sheltering woods.

Beth buried her face in her hands and shook for what seemed an eternity before she dared move. She gathered herself together and glanced at her compass. It swung weirdly, and her radio was emitting nothing but crackling static. Her instruments were useless. *There must be pig iron in this mountain.*

She was alone, without direction. She'd allowed herself to be coerced into depending on men she didn't know, and now she was part of the problem.

Panda nuzzled her cheek. *"Ve al carro,"* Beth begged. What was she thinking? How could she expect her dog to understand they needed to get back to the car? The shepherd studied her mistress's face, then trotted off.

Before long, a deep moonless night blanketed the forest. An owl hooted his presence behind them. Crickets chirruped, and frogs sang. Beth used her bandanna to tie her flashlight to Pan's neck and followed its wavering path.

It seemed forever before Panda led them into the illuminated tents of base camp. Beth flung her arms around her partner, almost smothering her. *"¡Perrita buena!"*

Panda shook free, swiped her mistress's hand with a wet tongue, and raced ahead of her downhill. "Wait for me. Wait for me."

The deputy leaned back in his camp chair and scratched his belly when he saw Beth. "You're back. We was going to send the crew out to look for you first thing."

"Tomorrow? It wouldn't be necessary if we'd stayed together. Did they arrive back here okay? No injuries?"

The deputy spewed a stream of tobacco juice, and Beth jumped out of range. "You had 'em leave their guns, remember? They was a little scared when they saw that bahr. But they're gonna go out and git that thing soon as it's light."

Beth remembered the beautiful creature who'd backed away in peace. "What bear? Is that why they ran?"

"You joshing me?"

"They'd be wasting their time. Did you find the hunter?"

"No, ma'am."

"Forget the bear, and let's think about finding him. Good night, Officer."

The hunter was discovered at sunup suffering from hypothermia. His body temperature had fallen so low that death had been only a matter of hours away. During the night he had taken off his wool shirt, wrapped it around a stick, and burned it like a torch. He had thought he might light his way home. He was wrong.

After this search, Beth believed she'd seen the limits of Panda's extraordinary talents. She, too, was wrong.

CHAPTER 6

INTELLIGENT DISOBEDIENCE

August 1985

The phone's ring pierced the predawn peace. Beth squinted in the early Saturday half light at digital numbers glowing a too-early 5:09 A.M. "Morning, Bob."

Panda was up immediately. A series of tiny whines betrayed that the shepherd recognized the name of the DOGS East dispatcher.

"Grayson National Forest? It'll take me hours to get down there. Aren't there any teams closer?" Beth listened. Indeed there were; but they had already been on the job a couple of days with no luck.

She watched her partner jump to the floor and pad silently out of the room. "Yeah, Bob, don't worry, we'll get there as soon as we can." She tipped the phone into its cradle as Panda trotted back to the bed. The dog had already pulled her shabrack from the closet where Beth kept her gear. She dropped the orange jacket—"Rescue" and a white cross emblazoned on it—atop the spread, and waited.

"Okay." Beth yawned.

Interstate 81 was empty, so Beth could let her mind run over the practicalities ahead. Weather forecast predicted another 90-degree day, ditto humidity, no wind. That meant very little difference between the victim's body temperature and the ambient air: harder for Panda to detect the scent.

It didn't help that Grayson National Forest was rife with rhododendron and those scimitar-like thornbushes for which Virginia was famous. Add a maze of swamps, and the resultant hungry mosquitoes, and they had the worst possible search conditions. Lovely way to spend a weekend.

Beth was surprised to see only Bob waiting for her at the designated meeting place.

"You'd left before I could get back to you. We found the guy," he apologized. "But, Beth, the oddest thing. We just got another SOS from a nursing home not thirty miles from here. An Alzheimer's patient has gone missing. The rest of the team left already. You can pass on this if you want."

Beth considered. She thought about the bees swarming over every patch of color; the ticks she'd have to extract out of Panda's hide, and her own; the thigh-high undergrowth of a Virginia forest; and the sweat already beading on her back. Then she thought of some poor, confused man lost in that same morass of wilderness.

"I'm here, Bob," she said. "Where's this nursing home?"

Beth parked her new Blazer in the shade of a drooping poplar. She let Panda out the back and automatically checked the buckles on the dog's shabrack. Not only did the white cross emblazoned on its side give notice that they were on a rescue mission; in the fall season, it might save the dog from getting shot by some overeager hunter.

Next Beth gathered her own equipment—red coveralls, pack, radio, water, machete, hard hat, and Panda's Frisbee. Together dog and mistress found their way to the sheriff's car.

The team leader for this mission was Marion Hardy, the same old friend who had joined Beth at Quantico for that first search three years ago. A kind, no-nonsense woman with a cap of prematurely gray hair and eyes of deepest cobalt, Marion, to Beth, was a kindred spirit.

"Glad you could make it." The woman smiled. "How much time can you spare?"

Beth appreciated Marion's focus because it mirrored her own. She calculated in terms of twelve-hour segments. "Three. I can leave no later than tomorrow afternoon."

"Search, sleep, search?"

"I'd rather do a straight twenty-four hours, then rest," Beth replied. "In this heat, Panda's got a better chance of picking up the scent at night."

"No problem. Our victim is a tall man of medium weight, suffering from diabetes and dementia. He's been missing a day and a night, so he's been without medication for a long time." The information was relayed with the crisp, precise brevity Beth had come to appreciate. "The staff at the home swear the man would never go off the road or into the bushes."

Why did people always say that? Beth thought.

The two women got out of the coolness of the air-conditioned car, and Marion unrolled her topo map. "I've deployed teams covering north and east. Let me see now. . . ." The team leader held her map on her knee and scanned the red-lined areas.

Beth shaded her eyes against the bright sunshine. Shimmers of heat hovered above the black tarmac of the driveway. It was going to be another killer day. She probed for movement in the yellow acres of cleared fields beyond, but nothing stirred on the exposed land.

It made sense to Beth that even an Alzheimer's patient would seek out a cooler place. She pointed toward a nearby mountain undulating within a blue-purple haze. "Has anyone gone that way?"

Marion looked up and frowned. "Our man's not supposed to be able to make it that far, but . . ." She considered. "Go for it, Beth. Keep in close radio contact. I'll have some of the local talent follow a couple of miles behind."

It was late afternoon before they reached the meadow near the top. Beth had stopped every twenty minutes to let Panda drink and rest. It was vital to keep a search dog well watered.

The settling relief of twilight surrounded them when they reached the higher levels. Panda wove in front of her mistress in her familiar, loping gait. Beth was beginning to think she'd been wrong in her assumption that the victim would seek cooler altitudes, but then no word had come that he had been found anywhere else.

Up ahead, the waist-high vegetation opened out into a grassy meadow. Panda trotted across the pasture to where a huge stand of blackberries rambled down toward a gentle drainage valley, forming an oval of thorn-to-thorn vines. The brambles were so thick Beth couldn't see through them, but Panda ran straight to their prickly edges. A flock of pheasants screeched in protest, and beat the air in retreat. Cicadas whirred in their rising and falling chant to the heat.

The dog's ears strained forward; then she swung around and dashed back to her mistress. Beth watched the alert in disbelief—the heat must have gotten to Pan. Nothing and nobody could be in that mess.

"No, *amiga*." She tacked a crosswise path to bypass the impenetrable thicket. "This way."

The shepherd parked herself directly in front of her mistress and bumped her toward the bushes. Beth was irritable and drained from the day's fruitless search. She knew Panda couldn't be feeling much better. "No, *perra*, no," she insisted.

Panda hesitated barely a second. She started at a trot; then her legs were pistons hurtling her body like an arrow for a full frontal attack on the copse.

"No!" Beth screamed, but too late. The thorns gripped the dog in their talons. The more Panda struggled, the deeper the needles embedded their pain into her body. "No, no, no!" Beth yelled.

She unsheathed her machete and slashed at the torturous bush that imprisoned her partner. The dog whined and thrashed. Beth forced her voice low, calming the shepherd—and herself. "*Mira. Mirame.* Look at me, Pan." Her friend turned toward her. Beth was distressed at the glazed look of torment in the familiar chocolate eyes. "*Calmate, mi perrita,*" she repeated until Panda stopped writhing.

Slowly, methodically, Beth cut and eased, cut and eased. She stomped her boots hard on the sinewy branches; the barbs tore at her face, but she felt nothing. It seemed to take forever before she could wrap her arms around Panda's body. "Hold on, girl." Beth braced and stepped back, wincing at the handfuls of white hair torn from the dog's body as she came free. She staggered and gently lowered her partner to the ground.

Panda's snowy fur was spattered with blood. Beth hurriedly opened her first-aid kit. "Shhh. Shhh," she soothed as she cleaned the wounds and anointed them with antibiotic. Pan whimpered quietly, but didn't move.

"Beth! Beth!" The voices came from four young men jogging their way uphill. "I'm Paul. I'm a vet tech with the rescue squad," said one, and knelt beside the dog.

But the shepherd would have none of it. Panda struggled to her feet and limped toward the blackberry patch. "She obviously knows something we don't." Beth sighed. "Do you have machetes? We're going to cut a passage for her."

And they did. For the next half hour, Panda was their operations leader. She'd wait behind as they attacked the heart of the brambles. When they stopped for breath, she'd move into the breach and let out a single, sharp cry. "Keep going," Beth ordered. Panda's muffled keening was their signal to slow down.

"Easy now, easy," Beth said. "Our man must be close." A few more feet and they found him. Spread-eagled on the bush, naked except for his underwear, he looked like he'd been flayed by a cat-o'-nine-tails. Punctures and scratches lacerated every surface of his body. Dried and fresh blood painted amazing patterns on his flesh. How had he ever gotten in so deep?

The victim was unconscious and in shock, and slipping quickly into a diabetic coma. The medics pried him loose and laid him on a stokes litter. They covered him with the thin blanket from their pack, then radioed for an ambulance to meet them at the fire road.

"We'd better carry Panda out, too," Paul insisted, as he and his friend hoisted the dog between them. In silent procession, the party started out from the thicket.

Beth couldn't relax until the patient was placed safely into an ambulance and Pan was checked by the vet tech. Luckily the shepherd was not badly hurt from her ordeal, and Beth was determined it would be more than mere Frisbee play for a reward this night.

"The thickest, juiciest burger I can find for you, young lady," she promised as she made Panda comfortable in the back of the Blazer for their drive home. "You saved that man's life."

For the five hours it took to get back to her house, Beth thought about the events of the day. This was the first time she'd faced anything worse than a sprained ankle—and the first time her dog had ever disobeyed an order.

Beth needed to think through the lesson of Panda's unusual behavior—this intelligent disobedience. Were there no limits to the shepherd's gifts?

At that moment Beth knew the answer was "no."

PART TWO

EARNING THE PATCHES

CHAPTER 7

DISASTER—
EL SALVADOR

San Salvador, El Salvador

On October 10, 1986, Atlas shrugged.

The resultant temblors were fifteen minutes apart, and measured 5.4 and 4.5 on the Richter scale—hardly enough to send a shiver up the spine of most Los Angelenos. But Atlas was careless. He picked a tiny corner of the world, trapped for decades in civil war, hunger, poverty, and corruption. There, his wavelets proved cataclysmic. Atlas chose El Salvador.

It was no ordinary call that disturbed the pleasant lassitude of Beth's Friday evening. She and Panda had passed all their evaluations; they were now "operational," a label for a professional SAR team. But the Virginia Department of Emergency Services was not asking for help in finding a missing person in the wilderness this night. The quest on which Beth Barkley and her Panda were about to embark would involve the Agency for International Development, the Office of Foreign Disaster Assistance, and the State Department, among others. It would affect the lives of not just a few, but thousands, of people.

"You might have seen on the news that El Salvador has experienced a devastating earthquake. The United States is sending aid immediately." The voice on the other end of Beth's telephone was brisk and to the point, as befitted a government official with a mission to accomplish. "OFDA has asked for four dog handlers to be at Andrews Air Force Base at 0300 hours. Your name was put forward. Understand that, if you agree, you will have to make arrangements to be gone for several days."

Her boss at AT&T would be reluctant to give her a leave of absence, but Beth had vacation time coming. She'd have to use it to go on this mission. *Oh, well, who needed a vacation anyway?* Three in the morning gave her and Panda plenty of time to get to Andrews. "I can make it, sir," Beth said. "Would you mind telling me who else will be on the team?"

The few seconds of silence was punctuated by the rustling of papers. "Bill Dotson will be your team leader. Two of the other handlers are Caroline Hebard and Phil Audibert. Both, like you, have the advantage of speaking Spanish. That gives us three of the four needed. We're considering whom to send as the fourth handler."

Bill and Phil were both from her group, DOGS East. She'd never worked with Caroline but knew her from conferences. Beth had an idea who might round out the foursome. "May I make a suggestion?"

"Go ahead."

"You might want to consider Heidi Yamaguchi. She doesn't speak Spanish, and she's still a trainee, but her dog Shiro is very good and small. He'd be able to get into places the other dogs might find difficult."

"We'll take it under advisement. And Ms. Barkley, please bring your passport."

Along with the other three handlers and their dogs, a "critical incident stress" psychologist, civil engineers, satellite communications specialists, and various and sundry State Department personnel, Beth climbed aboard the C-141 Starlifter. But it was only as they leveled off headed due south toward El Salvador that Beth began to realize the enormity of their mission.

CALLE RUBÉN DARÍO

Day 1: Saturday, October 11, 0800

The ponderous weight of the landing gear grumbled free of constraints as the belly of the military transport approached Ilopongo airfield. Beth wrapped her fingers tightly around the smooth armrest and tensed for landing. The smell of rubber burning, a sudden jolt, then blessed silence.

Nobody moved for a few seconds. A gray-suited man from an intelligence agency nobody named snapped open his seat belt. An aging State Department official eased stiffly out of his seat. One by one the thirty-five men and women who made up the U.S. humanitarian aid team shifted, stirred, and popped out the earplugs they'd been issued prior to takeoff.

Beth followed their example, and shook her head to dissolve the ringing that had seemingly taken up permanent residence inside her skull. But she was more concerned for Panda's ears. There had been no military equipment issued to protect the team's dogs against the monstrous barrage of noise. *"Está bien. Está bien,"* she murmured, kneading the soft fur and skin that was Panda's only protection for her precious hearing.

She knew the other three handlers would be doing much the same for their own dogs. She also knew they'd all have the same thought. *When will they open those doors and let us get our animals to some grass?*

The U.S. team waited, dividing into small groups, murmuring possibilities and tactics among themselves. Minutes passed. The rain-choked heat of the Salvadoran summer seeped relentlessly into the cavernous interior of the windowless transport aircraft. Sweat beaded the brows of those whose soft flesh betrayed their sedentary lifestyle. Others stretched and flexed, impatient with the delay.

Smiles of relief greeted the rolling grind of metal against metal that signaled the egg-domed door was sliding free. Everyone surged to the rear, blinking against the sudden, blinding clarity of sunlight.

That was as far as they got. On the empty tarmac below, a ragtag line of teenage soldiers waited, the ugly muzzles of their machine guns aimed directly at the Americans.

"Great," someone muttered.

It was no secret that the United States had taken the side of President Duarte in the vicious civil war that ravaged the tiny Central American nation. Everyone surmised that there were political as well as humanitarian reasons the United States was rushing aid to the stricken country.

At the 5:00 A.M. "in country" briefing before takeoff, the State Department official had addressed the issue directly. "The United States wants the Salvadoran people to know we are their friends, but in certain quarters

Americans are not welcome. A group of our marine boys were killed by leftists a couple of months ago.

"So you will only be allowed to move around in designated areas and under armed escort at all times. Now, we understand the guerrillas have called a cease-fire during the crisis. But don't count on it, and good luck."

Beth remembered those words as she stared down at their welcoming committee. The fourteen-year-olds were getting restless. One of the boys, taller than the rest, seemed to be fixated on Panda and Shiro. Beth recalled that in North America it was a common practice, in certain circles, to kill a white German shepherd at birth. Could the same superstition hold true south of the border? She and Heidi Yamaguchi both handled white German shepherds. The whip-crack precision of a safety being eased echoed in the deathly quiet, and Beth pulled Panda closer.

The Americans' attention was diverted by the turbo roar of motor engines. Charging toward them at loco speed were three ancient, armor-plated vehicles. One after the other they jolted to a halt between them and the boy soldiers. As the dust settled, a tall, bald-headed man jumped lightly down from the passenger side of the lead van.

In embarrassing contrast to the nervous, sweaty crowd staring down at him, he was a study in cool and immaculate. Café-au-lait skin and dark mustache were the handsome backdrop to the flawless crispness of a white guyabara shirt. Knife-edge creases lined his khaki slacks; tan loafers finished his casual outfit to perfection. One stern nod, and the Uzis were lowered. Satisfied, the savior turned his attention to the Americans.

"Welcome," he said, his dark eyes missing none of the smiles of relief. "I'm James. Alejandro James."

"He's one of ours," sighed the individual from the intelligence agency.

"*Sí.* OFDA. I am to be your liaison for the duration."

Beth liked the tall Panamanian right away, and not because he was one of the handsomest men she'd ever seen. He had heart. Beth knew it when he insisted all the dogs get some relief before they drove into the capital. On the way, she listened carefully to what he had to say.

"You must remember that San Salvador is a perpetual war zone. Guns, soldiers, snipers, bombs, these are our daily fare. Let us hope it is not yours."

"Now I know why Mom thought I was crazy to come here," Heidi whispered to Beth.

"You didn't know about the civil war?"

"Sure I did. I just didn't pay too much attention to it."

"We have made arrangements for you to stay at the Hotel Presidente downtown," Alejandro continued. "It is truly lovely. I can personally vouch for that."

Beth believed him. Alejandro gave the impression of a man accustomed to five-star accommodations.

"However, first we must go to Calle Rubén Darío. Five of your extrication specialists have already arrived from Miami. They are in need of your assistance."

"What is a Calle Rubén Darío?" Heidi inquired.

Alejandro took a few seconds before answering. "Now, unfortunately, it is a shambles. Before the earthquake it was a lovely complex of stores, clinics, restaurants, and offices." He paused. "We estimate there could be as many as twelve hundred people buried there."

A startled gasp was drowned by the grinding gears of the armored van.

* * *

Beth and the rest of the team were able to see for themselves what their liaison had been talking about as they came into the city. Block after block of the modern buildings that surrounded the squares so beloved of the *capitalinos* had pancaked into rubble. The shanties, cobbled together out of wood and tin, had fared rather better than their neighbors of concrete and steel. Beth couldn't miss the irony.

It concerned her to see men, women, and children sifting through the remains of their homes; any aftershock could swallow them alive. Others seemed to understand the danger. They'd set up camp on the sidewalks under tents of plastic trash bags, using scavenged pots to cook over shards of wood pulled from the surrounding wreckage. It was the old human imperative to protect territory—even if the territory was only a pile of rubble.

It was raining when they pulled into the Calle Rubén Darío—a short, drenching cloudburst Beth and her colleagues would become used to over the next six days. A vital bear of a man, sporting the blue fire-rescue uniform of the Florida team, was ensconced on a sidewalk under a big beach umbrella. "I'm Doug Jewett," he boomed. "Great, great, you got here. Go 'round the building and tell us where those mutts think the people are." The man was wasting no time in putting them to work, but Beth got the feeling Doug Jewett was less than thrilled at the presence of the animals.

They were to start at the Rubén Darío commercial building, which, at eight stories, had been the biggest on the street. The men from Miami, members of the Metro-Dade rescue squad, spoke fluent, street-wise Spanish. No fools, they'd enlisted the help of the local men to shore up the voids created between plumbing, doorways, concrete against concrete.

The four handlers removed the shabracks from their animals. When the dogs searched the collapsed rubble of buildings after a hurricane or earthquake, they always worked "nude." There was too much danger from reinforcement bars, jagged concrete, daggers of wood that could catch the orange jackets and injure the dogs.

They were to search in teams of two, each taking a turn to explore the newly excavated hole. When one handler-and-dog team finished, their teammates would go in to confirm any alerts. Beth was coupled with Caroline, whose male shepherd, Aly, preferred to work with a female dog; Heidi worked with Phil and his golden retriever, Matlock.

The gaping holes the men from Metro-Dade had assessed as being safe for them to enter would have given any sensible person pause. But from the beginning, Beth felt comfortable with their decisions. Their running repartee, spiced with earthy jokes in Spanish, made her smile. It didn't take a rocket scientist to guess they were aware of the volatile mood of the populace and were determined to keep things light.

Death and disaster of this magnitude were new to both dog and mistress, fraught with dangers that went a quantum leap beyond wild animals, drunken hunters, exhaustion, hypothermia, and other potential dangers of a wilderness search.

Beth was surprised she felt no fear. Panda led the way, as surefooted as if she were training on the rubble pile back home, showing her mistress the safe places to crawl forward. They were in a secret universe, the woman and her beloved *perrita*. The sullen crowds, hostility, war, and possibility of sudden death faded away in the focus on the job at hand.

There were people alive in this mess, Beth knew it. This was what she and Panda had trained and worked for for six long years. To save lives.

Panda slowed in front of her. The dog's square back tensed, her tail stiffened. Beth could faintly make out the quiver of a pink nose in the murky ambient light. Panda's big head butted against an overhanging slab of concrete and Beth scrambled to crouch beside her animal. This was not the slow pawing of a dead find. Panda sensed life close by.

"Hup, hup," Beth commanded with a smack on the ledge above them. Panda leaped into the darkness with the grace of a gymnast. Without hesitation she pushed up on her hind legs and Beth heard the light scratch of paws against metal. Some pipes blocked the shepherd's way. And behind that metal someone was *alive*.

"*Aquí, mi perrita. Ahora,*" she commanded, and Panda was immediately by her side. Beth marked the spot twice. Panda had alerted to death many times in the last few hours; now the shepherd's priceless olfactory scent cells were telling her mistress something different. Confirmation was needed. Immediately!

Fifteen minutes was all dog and handler were allowed inside the rubble. The rules were that you gave no indication of any find to your teammate's dog. Aly's alert had to confirm Panda's. Beth passed onto the street with a nod to Bill Dotson, and a small smile to the unruffled image of Alejandro James.

"This is no fun, is it?" he said, falling in beside her.

"Water and shade is the order of the hour, don't you think?" Alejandro waved aside a child guard and pointed across the banana curve of the street where Doug Jewett waited.

The man from Metro-Dade had done them proud. He'd moved their umbrella in front of the relative safety of AT&T's building; its stone, riot-proof first floor still stood. He'd also managed to scrounge a well-worn oblong table, of the type used by farmers to sell their produce in the open markets, and set three wooden chairs around it.

"Here ya go, Beth. Just for you and that worthless mutt. All the comforts of home . . . that is, if your home doesn't have electricity, running water, a toilet. . . ." The grin that split his tan Cuban-American face was meant to reassure.

"Boy, I thought you'd manage better than this," Beth teased. But Alejandro was too busy scratching the ears of Beth's "worthless mutt" to answer.

The shade was almost cool after the 110-degree stress of below ground. Panda belly-flopped to the pavement and lapped greedily at the clear water her mistress had poured into her bowl.

Beth could barely stand the waiting. Pan had alerted to somebody alive. Caroline and Aly should have confirmed it by now. What was taking them so long? Where were they? Someone was still breathing in that wreck of a building. She knew it.

She half-listened to Alejandro's answer to her question of why so many of the men between the ages of sixteen and fifty had an arm or leg missing.

". . . so you see, that's why all the guards are children.

SEARCH AND RESCUE   53

As soon as they're old enough to go fight, a land mine blows them up."

He shook his head, the charm of his smile wiped away by the bitterness of his recollections. Beth touched his arm in sympathy, then stiffened. Aly and Caroline had emerged.

"Excuse me, Alejandro," Beth said. "I'll be right back."

But Panda moved first. Her head shot up. A blur of white and she was off the sidewalk, and in the middle of the street.

"Pan, no," Beth shouted. What on earth was her dog doing? Panda whirled, stared, then hung her head as if in apology. *"Aquí,"* Beth commanded, slapping her thigh. But Panda didn't move. And Beth saw a warning that was to become eerily familiar in the days ahead. Panda's ears stood out flat, wide, straight out from her head, like rotors on a helicopter about to spin her away.

Beth ran toward her. *Trust your dog. Trust your dog.* The mantra of search and rescue pounded in her brain. Panda was trying to tell her something. But what? Underneath her feet the earth rumbled, throwing its bellyache upward. And Beth knew.

She threw herself on the ground. Around her men, women, and children screamed and shoved in panic as they scattered. On her periphery, Beth was dimly aware of the rasping scrape of concrete shifting, the whoosh of gravel and dirt imploding into itself.

The aftershock was only a few seconds; then the sky opened. A hot, torrential cloudburst rained down on the earth and its people as if to wash away the fears. Twenty yards away Heidi's eyes were wide in disbelief. Next to her, Phil had a firm grip on the muff of his gentle retriever.

But Caroline was talking to their team leader, her hand punctuating the air with sharp, rapid gestures, pointing to the collapsed building behind her. Bill Dotson listened without interruption, then took off at a run, shouting for the Metro-Dade men. Caroline grinned, bent over, twisting her long blond mane like a rope, squeezing the water from her hair.

"You all right?" Beth asked her teammate.

"Never better." Beth could *feel* Caroline's excitement. "Aly almost tore the flashlight out of my hand in there."

"Panda's ears and tail were up."

The two women were talking the language of search and rescue. Neither had to tell the other their dogs had alerted to a live find.

The message spread through the strike team, was called out to the men from Miami, and was picked up and passed, one excited word after another, through the crowd.

The *americano*s had found people alive.

The United States had the only search-and-rescue teams in San Salvador that first day. They worked sixteen straight hours, pushing themselves to the point of collapse. In the first day and a half, Metro-Dade brought out thirty-two people alive. Seven were the direct result of specific alerts by the four dogs. Many more were brought out because the canines had silently told the rescuers to keep digging—that in this place someone still clung to life.

WHITE TENNIS SHOES

Day Two: Sunday, October 12

"We need more help here, dogs, equipment. . . ." Bill Dotson's southern drawl had degenerated into terse frustration by Sunday morning. The U.S. team had realized they were understaffed as soon as they arrived. The two quakes had leveled the U.S. embassy and effectively cut off communication to the outside world.

"We could do with at least a half dozen more teams down here," the team leader complained, worrying that his people were fast becoming overwhelmed. The four dogs had been dragged from one search site to the next as desperate relatives swore they heard cries and poundings. If only the *americanos* would come and look, their loved ones would be saved.

"We need more dogs. . . ." Bill Dotson reiterated to the team, preaching to the choir.

His wish was soon answered. Unbeknownst to him, an SOS had resounded around the world. Before the Americans had finished sharing their lunch of cheese and bologna sandwiches with some of the famished street urchins at the barricades, the foreign contingents descended.

The Swiss arrived first. They marched into the Calle Rubén Darío, a moving platoon of orange uniforms, dogs tightly leashed beside them, more military than the military. The French, Dutch, Italians, and British followed. Before it was over, teams from fourteen nations swarmed like bees upon the nectar of one tiny country's disaster.

Now another kind of frustration threatened to overwhelm the rescuers—coordination. The precarious ruins of downtown regressed into towers of babel and bark.

Bark? Back home, one of the unwritten tenets of wilderness search is that no well-trained dog alerts with a bark. That alone does not indicate if the victim is dead or alive. Worse, a barking dog could terrify a lost child or older person in the bush.

The handlers from the United States forged intense, passionate bonds with their working partners that went far beyond those normally found in the people/pet relationship. The stateside dogs all had their own particular ways of communicating with their "persons," and Beth and her teammates had come to understand every nuance of their animals' body language. To know the difference between their dog's alert on a possible live find and a dead person was crucial. If dead, the spot would be noted and tagged, but not immediately excavated. If someone might be alive, the work of rescue would begin at once. Panda's animated response, as contrasted to her subdued reaction, was literally a matter of survival or death.

Not so with the European dogs. These canines yowled at blood, body fluids, body parts, any and all possibilities. The American team couldn't believe what they heard.

But it was the sheer numbers of dogs, handlers, and auxiliary personnel all trying to work together that roiled frustrations.

As far as Beth was concerned, the Swiss were impossible. Everywhere she turned it seemed orange uniforms cut above, in front, or around her, showering pebbles of concrete, or shifting the unstable pile in their wake. "Brunhilde," the nickname the Americans bestowed on the tall, Wagnerian female who dogged their search areas, was the flash point.

Beth felt sorry for the woman's dog. A beautiful golden, the size of a small sheep, the animal was aggressive toward the other dogs yet seemed bewildered by the noise and cowed by his mistress's harangues. Late in the afternoon, he had reached his limit.

Brunhilde was poised over a newly excavated hole. She dropped to her hands and knees and peered into the void. Seemingly satisfied, she stood and uttered the guttural words of command for her dog to go forward.

The retriever tentatively picked its way to the very edge of the hole and looked down its sloping darkness. He recoiled, slunk onto his belly, and sank his golden head into his paws.

Take him out of here. Can't you see he's had enough? Beth wished she dared speak to the woman.

Then Brunhilde did the unforgivable. She inhaled three loud breaths, bent, slid her muscular arms under her dog's belly and hoisted him skyward. A bright flush infused the points of her cheeks as she staggered like a drunk under the load. A grunt, a mighty heave, and Brunhilde slung the poor beast around her neck and grabbed his paws. The woman looked like some prehistoric hunter coming in with her kill.

The Swiss handler caught the stares of the watching Americans. A sneer creased her blunt features. She bent and maneuvered the limp animal into a more comfortable position across her shoulders. With Germanic determination, Brunhilde marched both of them into the abyss.

Enough. Enough of this. *"Ven conmigo, Panda."* Beth ordered, and led them carefully off the west side of the building to the sidewalk.

State Department personnel and their counterparts with the Swiss team were already conferring. The Americans would be trucked to other locations while the decision-makers sorted out how to keep their rescuers out of each other's way.

The U.S. team fumed in the stifling heat of the armored van. The Rubén Darío was easily the hardest hit; that was where they should be concentrating their efforts, not elsewhere.

"Would you pass that up front, please?" The request came from the embassy guard riding shotgun. He nodded at the floor beneath Heidi's feet.

The handler thrust her hands under her seat and pulled out a menacing-looking Uzi. "Is this loaded . . . sir?"

"Sure hope so, ma'am. You'll find another one right behind it, if you don't mind."

It hadn't fazed Beth to be surrounded by Latinos toting machine guns; she'd somehow expected it. But the easy nonchalance of one of their own with such a weapon brought home once again the reality of their situation.

The van lurched to a halt, and the handlers cautiously followed each other into the bright sunshine.

They were in another square, this time a market square. It was beautiful, faced on one side with a park filled with the fuchsia hues of bougainvillea. The jagged ruins of buildings curved like the broken handle of a cup. Sidewalks steamed with fresh rain.

Their assigned building had once stood five stories above the street; the earthquake had settled it one full story into the earth. Now its jumbled remains rested like a clutch of broken Lego blocks on the sidewalk.

The *capitalinos* moved back as the team single-filed

behind their guard. Beth had become used to the intent watch of the throngs that had crowded the barricades at Calle Rubén Darío. She'd sensed no malice in their curiosity. The children appeared fascinated with the dogs, and always wanted to touch them.

"¿Son bravos, los perros?" they would ask. "Do they bite?" Beth had translated for Heidi. She would take the hands of the child who'd ventured the question, and guide them over first Panda's and then Shiro's head. *"No."*

"Seems we're home safe with our white dogs," Heidi had whispered.

"Maybe," Beth had murmured. But inwardly she was pleased. *"Buena, Panda, perrita de mi corazòn,"* She would croon her favorite term of endearment to the elegant dog who nuzzled the marveling children. These had been moments of respite in the bleakness of loss.

But in this marketplace Beth felt hostility. She saw no smiles on the faces they passed. She sensed something she couldn't define in the attitude of the watchers.

They attacked the back of the building first, Heidi sending Shiro up a ladder in a show of agility. Nothing. Slowly they worked their way over the jumble of concrete and metal, navigated the obstacle course of sudden holes and collapsed tunnels, vertical chutes and horizontal voids, shards of glass dense as a carpet, piercing as rapiers to the unwary.

The dogs' alerts were subdued. There were no survivors here. The clouds massed thick and heavy in the tropical afternoon, the rains threatening to drench them yet again. The team decided to go back to the sidewalk to wait it out.

Phil's golden retriever Mat was as big as Panda and calm in nature. Mat and Phil had achieved the intense rapport that comes with years of an animal/person working team. So when Mat suddenly turned and led his master back to the broken edge of a pancaked balcony, everybody paused.

The big, tawny animal was pawing and sniffing in a most peculiar fashion. Phil squatted beside his dog, puzzled. "What is it, boy?" The three women moved closer. Beth dropped to her knees beside her teammate. In the street, the belligerent crowd nodded at each other and pressed forward. The *americanos* had found somebody.

Phil and Beth couldn't see anything at first, but Mat's alert was insistent. The retriever didn't recoil, as was his habit when the find was dead. Yet there was no furious blur of tail, no ears perked up like a startled rabbit's. Mat was giving none of his reliable signals for life.

Then Beth saw her. The dark-skinned woman must have run for shelter when the quake hit and crouched under the overhanging balcony, thinking she'd be safe. She'd made a fatal mistake. She'd been partially crushed and may have died only a short time before.

Phil had spied her, too. He stood and signaled for Caroline and Heidi to join them, and the four handlers hunched together to discuss Mat's find. None of them saw what went on behind them; they heard the murmuring first, a growing wave of sound ominous in its intensity. But this time it wasn't an aftershock. What the handlers were hearing was the rising anger of a people on the edge.

In the front of the crowd a man raised a fist. Other clenched hands lifted to the sky. A mob mentality was taking hold.

The Americans backed up, calling their dogs. Phil

turned. "Mat, Mat come. . . ." His words slipped into nothingness.

His retriever stood framed like a gilded statue against a crystalline sky, leg raised. A stream of urine sprayed onto a tumble of broken bricks. Mat was telling his master that he'd found a person, but she didn't smell right. Or perhaps it was the effect of two days of finding so many humans he considered part of his pack, dead under his nose. Mat was a dog. This was his natural way of expressing emotion. But to the angry rabble closing in on them, it was a rabid act of disrespect.

Their American guard, his Uzi high, finger on the trigger, backed toward them. "Aw, shit," said the young American with the buzz cut.

Caroline turned and shouted at the crowd. *"El perro . . ."*

Beth repeated her words in English for the benefit of Phil and Heidi. "The dog has found this poor woman, and is showing how upset he is by marking her. He must feel a kinship with her to show such a sign of respect."

"Sí, sí, es verdad," Beth yelled back at her colleague. It was indeed true. The dog was showing his sadness and respect.

The mob hesitated, surprised at the American women's fluent Spanish. Caroline and Beth continued the affirmations of respect, allowing Phil to grab Mat and steer him in a zigzag path out of sight. Heidi and Shiro disappeared next. Beth, Caroline, and their guard brought up the rear. They hit the corner and kept going.

It was when they'd made it through the market and were congratulating themselves on their escape that Phil asked the question. "Do you think the rebels were inciting that crowd? How can you tell who's a leftist and who's not?"

Their guard didn't break stride. "The guerrillas wear white tennis shoes."

Nobody said anything as they hiked to safety. *Everybody* wore white tennis shoes.

It had not been a winning day. The team arrived back downtown to be told that from then on the United States would divide their efforts on the Rubén Darío with the Swiss. Each would work four hours, then allow their counterparts to take over. Even the one bright spot of the morning for Beth had no closure. Five hundred people had been buried in the rubble of the office building attached to the presidential palace. But Panda had shown her mistress more clearly than the sun that burned their eyes that at least one was alive. Caroline and Aly confirmed, but it would take hours to ascertain if a rescue had been made. Beth could only hope that the local civil engineer who'd been with them would keep his promise and let them know.

The Americans dragged themselves back to their hotel after another grueling day of search and sometimes rescue. The Hotel Presidente was a walled extravaganza, frequented by rich travelers. Amazingly, the only damage was a foot-wide crack the length of the swimming pool. None of the strike team felt comfortable coming from the garbage-strewn streets peopled with *capitalinos* who had lost everything, to a five-star residence complete with chef.

The staff warned the handlers not to take their dogs to the front of the building to relieve themselves—*you will get kidnapped or killed. Stay in the garden, you will be safe there*. The luxury inside the walls was surreal against the reality of misery and death the Americans witnessed on the streets.

Yet it was blessed relief to take a shower. And the U.S. team found a unique way of cleaning their uniforms; they dropped them into their bathtubs and shuffled, jumped, and stirred them around underfoot, allowing the fresh, pine-fragrant suds of soap and water to wash away the sweat and pressures of the day. Beth shared with Panda the pleasure of the bath.

Dog and mistress were tired to the marrow when they finally fell into bed. But Beth's sleep was shallow, disturbed by the spasmodic bursts of gunfire beyond the outer walls.

CAUGHT IN THE VOID

Day Three: Monday, October 13

The peppery, sickly sweet, fetid odor came at them in waves when they returned to Rubén Darío the next morning. A common stench when bodies are reduced to a smear between collapsed concrete.

"Phew! Enough to knock you off your bloody feet, mate." The baby-faced Brit held his thumb and forefinger over his nose with a choice expression that said it all.

"Knock it off, Pete. We all got noses," a teammate shot back.

The British team had aligned themselves with the Americans within an hour of their arrival. They were a jolly band of four young men, whose obvious kinship with their dogs was as strong as that of their U.S. counterparts.

Beth didn't see the Brits tie up their dogs and ignore

them while they waited to search. She didn't see the Brits' dogs barking and snarling at any unfortunate who came near. The Englishmen petted, watered, and talked to their partners as if they were family. Which, of course, they were.

And Beth felt almost maternal about short, solid Peter. He seemed to go the extra yard when it came to taking care of Shep, his Border collie.

Early in the afternoon the Brits and the Yanks were dispatched to the Gran Hotel San Salvador. The hotel had been closed for renovations, with only an office in use by the American owner. But that still left the first-floor boutique emporium. Anywhere in the world, where there were shops, there were people shopping.

Beth and Peter flopped down under the shade of a corner porch across from the hotel to wait their turn to search. The cloying humidity of the tropics, the rot of garbage and decay, sapped their energy. Neither man nor woman felt like making conversation. Except to their dogs.

The Englishman dribbled water over his collie's head, murmuring softly to the heavy-coated animal. "Sorry, girl. I had to do it, you know."

"Why did you say that?"

"Say what?"

" 'Sorry' to Shep."

"Oh." Peter tried to smile. "Well, you see, our little island has a law that all dogs have to go into six months' quarantine if they leave the country. It's to prevent them bringing rabies back. We don't have rabies in England, you know."

"Six months! But you're on a humanitarian mission. Can't they make an exception?"

Peter shrugged and continued to cool his dog. "It's the

only way of making sure the animal doesn't have it, short of killing 'em. But Shep and me been together a lot of years now. I'm gonna hate to lose her."

"What are you talking about?"

The young man locked his elbows around his knees. "I haven't got the money. The government charges you to quarantine. I can't afford it. They'll put her to sleep when we get back."

"But . . . but . . . why did you bring her here?"

He looked up, surprise sharpening the round planes of his baby face. "How many lives have we saved? Besides, I'm part of the team. I can't let my team down."

Beth turned away. Saving lives was why she was there, too. And she understood about being part of the team. But what a price this young man would pay. She suddenly wished she wasn't just a working woman whose every spare penny went to her own animals.

"Isn't there anything . . . ?"

"I think it's your turn to go in." Peter nodded toward the Gran. Bill Dotson was beckoning her over.

Peter's confidence upset Beth. Now she was as morose as Panda. Beth had watched her dog's growing depression the past three days. Panda showed none of her affectionate playfulness when it was reward time; there was no wagging tail, no joyous bark of release when the day's job was done. And there was something Beth had never seen before. Panda refused to eat. She'd only downed one meal since they'd arrived. Beth had coaxed, cajoled, even tried to hand-feed her big, white baby—but Pan would have none of it.

The shepherd was used to finding dead people. Beth could only surmise it was the sheer number of bodies and body parts that was causing her to curl into herself, even when sleeping. And Beth's own growing frustrations couldn't be helping any either.

"At least I won't have to put you down when we get home," she muttered as she crawled behind her partner in the darkness.

The air pressed in on them, suffocating as they squeezed forward. Beth switched on the miner's lamp that banded her helmet, and a pale beam pierced the gloom. The sour odor of stagnant water offended her nostrils. She had a sudden insight of what it must be like to work underground for a living. "Poor sods," she muttered, unconsciously borrowing one of Peter's colorful expressions.

Up ahead, Panda paused and waited for her to catch up. Her partner had found an elevator shaft, sheared at the floor, jammed at a 90-degree angle. If they could burrow their way along its length toward the offices, they might find the American owner.

Dog and mistress wound upward. Twisted plumbing pipes became as threads in a maze to lead them back. The partners pushed on. They sloshed through ribbons of water. A slab of carrera marble torn from the lobby floor became a slide. Then Panda whined softly and alerted to someone dead straight above them. Something was dripping. Thick, wet, sticky. Blood—old blood, mingled with the relentless rain of the tropics—puddled darkly onto the back of the white shepherd.

They had found the American.

A piece of reinforcement bar ("rebar") speared the belt loop of Beth's brown slacks as she scrambled toward daylight. It slowed her exit, leaving her a few seconds behind Panda out of the Gran Hotel.

Déjà vu greeted her. Another mob pushing against another barricade across another street, muttering, pointing, shaking their heads. Only the guns of the Salvadoran guards keeping them at bay. *What's the matter this time?*

"Beth." Heidi's soft voice wavered. She was thirty steps down the sidewalk, Shiro pulled tight against her side. Panda stood next to them, head down, fur starkly white against the blood staining her back and shoulders.

"Sangre! Sangre!" the crowd chanted. *Blood. Blood.*

Beth ran toward her teammate. "Water. We must wash Panda. God knows what these people are thinking."

Heidi immediately tore her canteen from her belt, opened it and poured, rubbing frantically. This seemed to incense the watchers even further, and Beth remembered that water was in scarce supply. And here were the Americans pouring it over a dog.

But Heidi was right. More and more their dogs had become goodwill ambassadors. People smiled as they passed, children petted them when they were allowed, giggled when the animals responded with wagging tails.

It had to be the blood.

A statuesque blonde ducked under the stiff-arm resistance of a guard, staggering under the weight of a five-gallon water jug. Beth recognized the woman; it was Janice Elmore, from the State Department. Janice wobbled toward her.

"Take this," she said, easing the glass container to the ground. "I'll see what I can do. Don't break it," she called as she loped away. "It belongs to the embassy. It's the last one."

Heidi nodded, frantic. She struggled to lift the jug, clasping her arms around its fat middle as if it were a sack of potatoes. She heaved it to her chest, and tilted. Water gushed over the white shepherd and ran off her back in bloody rivulets. Panda spread her legs, tensed, and shook her big body. A fine spray of pink rain showered over the women.

Heidi jumped back. Her fingers slid, lost their grip. "Help," she cried. The jug slipped further, aquamarine glass catching the sun, glinting like a precious stone, until it crashed onto the sidewalk in a craze of crystal pieces.

A river of water flowed over the curb, into the street. Silence.

"I think this is where we get out again," Beth said.

She grabbed Panda's ruff and edged slowly in the opposite direction from the stunned mob, down the long pavement between them and the other end of the building, to the armored van Bill Dotson had made their headquarters for this search.

Nobody stopped them.

The Brits took over for a while. Beth was too edgy to sit and rest. The crowd seemed to have forgotten the white dogs, concentrating their attention on the hole that led inside the Gran Hotel. Beth and her teammates watched and waited with them. Panda was restless, prowling around her mistress, nudging into her hand.

"Panda, tranquila," Beth soothed. *"Sientate."*

But Panda didn't sit. She cocked her big head, and for the fifth time in three days, took off to the emptiness of the street.

"One's a-coming," Beth warned, and the team scrambled into the street to join its lookout.

The earth shuddered as though an army of Hell's Angels, Harley throttles jammed open, had thundered down the street. A scattershot of jittery gunfire from the guards at the barricades was a prelude. Then the tremor hit.

Vehicles shook. *Capitalinos*, guards, Yanks, and Brits were slammed to the ground. The earth seemed to roll like waves. Debris, metal, the plants that had adorned an erstwhile balcony, glass, furniture, stone—crashing, re-aligning, finding new places to settle among the ruins of the Gran Hotel. Beth threw her arm over Panda and held on until it was finished.

People got up slowly. Everybody looked around, shock still frozen on their faces. Handlers ran their hands over their dogs and themselves, an automatic check to see if anything was broken. The complaining, muttering, weeping citizens were silenced.

Two Englishmen and three dogs picked themselves up, inches from the hole that branched into the twisted caverns of the once-grand interior of the Gran Hotel. They looked amazed to find they weren't crushed by falling rubble. But five men and four dogs had struggled inside. Three people and one animal were deep in that teetering building.

They're with us. We hooked up together. This can't happen. Beth read the same feeling in the faces of her fellow Americans. It was not because their governments decreed they should work together; not because they shared the same ideology; not even because the Brits and the Yanks trained their dogs in the same spirit.

It was simply that they were on the same side now, working together in a life-and-death situation, each scared one of the team might be injured, maimed— killed. *This can't happen.* Then Beth knew. Peter and Shep were inside.

Language is not always necessary to convey an emotion. The eyes of five hundred fixated as one on the dark, empty void.

A crack of wood splintered the silence, the rattle of a last dribble of gravel. The crowd held its collective breath. The quiet was unreal, the fear palpable.

But on this day, Atlas relented. Dust rose thick and gray from the void. Then, out of the cloud of debris, Shep ambled into the daylight. Peter and his teammate staggered into the street behind her, the arms of the third Brit wrapped around their shoulders.

The crowd sighed. Someone clapped. Peter grinned and threw up a "V" for victory. The watchers cheered.

The Yanks ran to their counterparts from across the ocean.

"Don't you do that again," Beth chided Peter, shoving him in the chest before she hugged him. "Nor you, Shep," she said, including the collie in her relief.

"Try not to, ma'am." Peter suddenly squatted beside his collie and held the quiescent dog's great head against his chest. Beth knew he was keeping back tears; her own eyes were moist. "Not Shep's time yet, anyway."

Peter realized what he'd said. "I didn't mean . . ."

"I know," Beth said quickly. "Let's get some water for her, shall we?"

Over their vehement protests, it was voted that the Brits should take the rest of the day off. The Yanks carried on. The days seemed to be getting longer with each hour. There was more gunfire that night. Panda didn't flinch. Beth thought she was dreaming.

THE PLACE OF THE UNBORN

Day Four: Tuesday, October 14

Alejandro was waiting for Beth and Panda the next morning. "The vice president of Costa Rica would like you to have breakfast with him," he said, matching her steps across the courtyard.

He was immaculate as ever, the white of his guyabara shirt dazzling in the early sunlight. Beth was acutely aware that she looked as crumpled as an old dollar bill. She saw Panda circle a square of earth in the garden, then hunch down her hindquarters. Beth stopped and tugged a plastic bag from her pants pocket. She grasped the bottom seam in her right hand and pulled the transparent material inside out back over her wrist.

"Why does he want to see me, Alejandro? What about the rest of the team?"

"He would like to meet all of you. But you're the first up this morning. You get to eat breakfast."

"Do I have to?"

"It might be good public relations for your country."

"Hold on a minute." Beth scooped up Panda's waste in the plastic, pulled the open end of the bag back over her hand, and tied the pouch closed.

"You do that very well," Alejandro noted, smiling.

"Lots of practice."

* * *

Breakfast was under a tree on the patio. Beth disposed of Panda's morning ablutions in a trash basket on the way to a table set with starched linen and silver. A feast awaited them: fruits, croissants, samovars steaming with coffee, eggs poached individually, served in round metal cups and wrapped with napkins.

Beth made no comment. She shook hands with the vice president, a short, cultivated individual, and dropped her knapsack on the ribbon of grass bordering the bank of flowers beside them. *"Con mis cosas,"* she murmured to Panda, and the dog obediently settled her elegant self beside her mistress's belongings.

"Your dog is very well trained," the vice president opened the conversation.

"Gracias," Beth replied.

"Did you know the Calle Rubén Darío is named after a famous South American poet?" Alejandro asked. They were back in the ubiquitous armored van on their way downtown.

"No," Beth answered quietly. She didn't feel like talking. Alejandro picked up her mood, and they rode the rest of the way in silence. "Best of luck, today," he murmured when the van stopped.

Beth nodded and let Panda onto the sidewalk. She allowed herself a few seconds to assess the familiar crumpled buildings, the stoic, watching faces of the gathered crowd, the orange uniforms of the Swiss lined up like a platoon on a far corner.

She wondered whether her reticence this day was because she had a gut hunch where they were to search:

the prenatal clinic. Rumor was that many had perished inside that building. But Beth was thinking of the perversity of life; some women conceived so easily, while she herself had failed so miserably. She pushed the jumble of thoughts and fears away, and disciplined her focus back to the mission.

Her guess had been right. When she reported for duty, her team leader led her a few steps out of earshot of any inquisitive listeners.

"We found a lot of bodies piled one on top of the other in there." He grimaced. "All we've had time to do is cover them with tarps. You'll have to crawl over them. You okay with that?"

Beth was okay with that.

"You know it's the prenatal clinic? I don't think any of the locals will go with you this time."

"Place of the unborn," Beth murmured.

"What?"

"Nothing."

Panda picked her way with care, placing one paw in front of the other, assessing the stability of her foothold before moving forward. The shepherd slunk low, teetering here and there as a paw sought unsteady purchase on a face, a shoulder, a foot. Beth crawled after her partner, wondering for the millionth time what emotions were running through the dog. Had she, like her mistress, numbed herself into a trancelike mission mode, with only one focus—to go forward? Or was the professional search dog nursing grief at the feel of so many of her "human pack" dead beneath her paws? Panda could never tell her in language. But this was her third day of refusing to eat. Before long they had passed over the tarped bodies and into the obscurity of another inward corridor.

Beth felt almost at home in these pockets of eternal shadows. She stood and tugged the miner's light lower on her forehead, following the beam's sweep around the space that had suddenly opened to them like a secret cavern. Twisted metal shelves clung to the ruins of walls. The surface beneath them was slick, shiny with hundreds of metallic wheels spilling reels of tape around the dim interior. A sign swung on one screw; "Sonogram Storage," it proclaimed in Spanish. They had found the prenatal clinic.

Deep rumbling—the earth itself moaned—and Beth braced for a tremor. The building groaned as if alive. Heavy friction caused metal supports and concrete slabs to screech in protest, and dust fell in sheets. Beth didn't want to die here.

Panda was calm. When the earth stilled, she turned dark eyes on her mistress, waiting for her order. Beth could only nod, and the dog explored again.

Something compelled her to do it. Her hands picked up first one, then another of the grimy wheels. She cleaned a section of tape with her thumb, staring as if it held the secrets of the universe. But Beth knew it told the stories of babies in the womb, and that up ahead lay the examination rooms for the women who'd carried them in their bellies.

The past slapped her in the face, worse than the aftershock they had just ridden out. So many years she'd tried to conceive. So much bitter medicine injected, swallowed, forced into herself. So many operations endured for the baby she desperately wanted. And all had failed.

This was a part of the woman kept hidden, unexamined. But now . . .

Her knees buckled and she fell. Beth Barkley rocked back and forth, sobbing into the darkness where nobody could hear, crying for the dead fetuses, for their mothers . . . and for her own shattered hopes.

She'd heard other rescue workers speak of this kind of reaction. She'd heard that they all at some time got hit by something. It may be the same thing they saw yesterday; but suddenly a sight, a sound, a motion, outside or inside them, would trigger a different response—and they would come undone. Sometimes right then, sometimes later. Now it was her turn, and she couldn't stop crying.

Warm breath caressed her wet face, and stiff, white fur scratched her cheek. "Panda, oh Panda," Beth cried, and flung her arms around her best friend.

She wanted to get out, get away. She crawled until the sunlight blinded her, and she gladly stumbled toward it. She stood, feeling almost indecently exposed under the naked sky.

A figure in a blue fire-rescue uniform walked quickly to her side. "Lean on me," the man from Metro-Dade murmured. Carlos Castillo cupped her elbow, and steered her toward the curb. "You need to sit down, Beth."

He waited like a silent sentinel while she sat, head in her hands, coiled into herself. "I just need fifteen minutes."

"You want to tell me what's the matter?"

Beth looked up into dark eyes calm with understanding. This man with the gleam of sweat on his mellow Caribbean skin had seen it all before. He knew without having to comprehend the details. Just his presence made her stronger.

"I'm okay now. I'm going back inside."

"Take your time. It's your call." He touched her shoulder in tacit empathy, and Beth was comforted.

For some reason she slept in oblivion this night, the first full rest Beth had managed since they'd arrived. She felt able to tackle anything when she awoke.

LA GORDA

Day Five: Wednesday, October 15

Doug Jewett was smiling this morning. "The powers that be have decided we're in charge now," he announced. Doug didn't bother to reveal who had performed this miracle, and he didn't have to explain that the orange Swiss uniforms would now have to follow the rules like everybody else.

Beth grinned at the solid Cuban-American. Metro-Dade had been the first on the scene when this disaster struck. They'd toiled for five days, only breaking for needed sleep and sustenance. Tomorrow the U.S. team would be going home. It was right this last day should belong to the men from Miami.

She saw Peter and Shep at the far end of the square next to the cathedral. The French, Belgian, and Dutch teams flanked the other side of the street. Back and forth came the shouts of many languages, the fractured interpretation, and the laughter as the relief of tensions floated in the air. Even the guards seemed more relaxed, allowing the handlers to lead their dogs at will to the barricades in order to be fussed over and petted by the *capitalinos*.

A feeling of camaraderie infused the plaza; the last communal effort was under way. Suddenly Beth felt full of energy. It was going to be a good day. Later she would be told that Panda's alert on a live person trapped in the pancaked ruins of the office building next to the Presidential Palace had been confirmed. "La Gorda" was the laughing nickname given to the victim by the Mexican miners who'd effected her rescue. She was a woman of massive proportions, over 300 pounds; it had taken thirteen hours to get her out. When everyone panicked and ran as the quake hit, she couldn't get her bulk up fast enough. The chair had skidded and got stuck in the frame of the door that led out of the office. That quirk of fate had saved her.

"She had two broken legs, but she was the only survivor in that whole building." The engineer, true to his word, had come back to report.

By curfew that night, five days into the rescue operation, all that any dog or handler could do was to indicate where the remains of what had once been human flesh and blood lay buried. The American team had almost forgotten the early successes of bringing out people alive. "La Gorda" reminded them that their mission, with all its stresses, had been worthwhile. Many were alive because they had come.

Two months later Beth received a thank-you letter. The sender had enclosed a newspaper photograph of Panda. The dog was framed in all her elegant whiteness, body stretched like a gymnast's, jumping into the black void that had led to "La Gorda."

GOING HOME

Day Six: Thursday, October 16

George Shultz had arrived.

The Secretary of State had flown in to survey the damage and reinforce the humanitarian presence of the United States. But it was the last few hours in Salvador for the strike team—their last chance to help the people of this country.

"You gotta be kidding!" someone exclaimed when told the secretary was on his way to meet with them.

"Let him have his picture taken with someone else."

"We still got work to do here."

Beth agreed with the grumbling. It wasn't that they didn't understand that the secretary had his work to do, too; it was just that everybody would rather have spent their precious remaining time on their own mission.

Secretary Shultz looked strained to Beth. He stood at the far end of Calle Rubén Darío, surrounded by men in dark suits. Their eyes roamed the assembled populace like foxes scanning a field for prey. Beth idly wondered if their suits were summer weight. Probably not. It was fall back in Washington. These guys would be sweating before the hour was over.

The Americans lined up. One by one they shook hands with the secretary, answered a question or two, and passed on. Finally, it was Beth's turn. "Good morning, Mr. Secretary," she murmured as she held out her hand.

The senior representative of the U.S. government didn't have a chance to answer. Beth felt Panda's belly heave against her leg, and heard her gag. Panda strained forward and with one huge gasp vomited a jaundiced, yellow mess over the spit-shined shoes of the secretary of state.

George Shultz barely hesitated. A quick glance downward, and he framed his question to the young woman in front of him.

"What is DOGS East?" he inquired, looking at the insignia on Beth's helmet. He had the bluest eyes. And he was trying hard not to laugh.

"We are a volunteer search-and-rescue group, sir." Beth jerked gently on Panda's leash to pull the shepherd behind her. "Three handlers, myself, and our dogs came with the U.S. team last Saturday, sir." Her foot skimmed the grass, scuffing up against the secretary's. Beth heard an ominous "squish" as her boot mashed the moist mess away. George Shultz didn't flinch.

"We're glad you came," he said, and grasped her hand. "We won't forget." The secretary couldn't hold it any longer. His professional formality dissolved into a big grin.

"Thank you, sir. And"—Beth glanced downward—"sorry."

"Don't give it another thought."

It was time to go. But first there were good-byes to be said. They crowded around each other, the Europeans and the Yanks, for once allowing their emotions release; hugs that lasted long seconds, promises to keep in touch, a tear here and there that flowed free.

The only one missing was Peter. Where was the boy?

"Beth." His unmistakable accent cut through the hum of farewells. She turned and saw the Brit running toward her, his bounding, furball of a dog panting alongside him.

A sadness wiped the smile from her face. Next to

Panda, Shep was the sweetest dog she'd ever worked with. It wasn't fair.

"I'll ask our liaison to help with Shep; we'll—"

Peter grabbed her hand. "Now listen up," he interrupted. "Somebody told the press here about Shep. How I didn't have the money for quarantine and all that. Well it seems one of our tabloids picked up the story and splashed it all over the front page. Talk about embarrassing." He grinned like a truant schoolboy. "But you know the Rolling Stones?"

Beth nodded impatiently. Who hadn't heard of the English rock stars?

"Charlie Watts, their drummer, called in and said 'no way.' Whatever it cost, no way was my dog to be put down just because of some rigid law. He's footing the whole bloody bill."

Now it was Beth's turn. She flung her arms around her friend's shoulders, whooping and laughing at the same time.

"Peter, Peter, Peter."

"It's absolutely terrific, isn't it? Shep's gonna go home with me. I'll visit her every day, see if I won't."

"Peter, I'm so, so happy for you."

"I know, luv. I knew you would be."

Sometimes there was justice in the world, Beth thought as the van took the Americans through the lush countryside of this beautiful tropical land. She doubted she would ever see her British friend again, but the memory of him and his beloved Shep would remain with her forever.

It was a very proper way to say good-bye.

CHAPTER 8

A STAR IS BORN

It had been seven months since El Salvador. Seven months of correspondence and telephone calls. Seven months visiting breeders to find another dog suitable for search-and-rescue work.

"It's like being pregnant . . . in the brain," Beth muttered as she picked up the phone to dial yet another lead, this one in Ontario, Canada. Joanne Chanyi had a twenty-five-year reputation for breeding the finest white German shepherds in North America.

"Hello?"

Beth felt nervous, excited, and apprehensive all at once. "Is this Joanne Chanyi?"

"This is she."

"My name is Beth Barkley, and I'm looking for a puppy."

"Yes, Beth. I've heard of you. You work with a white German shepherd." Joanne's voice was both cordial and friendly, and Beth released a soft sigh of relief.

"Her name is Panda. She's getting on eight years old."

"Hip dysplasia?" Joanne asked, referring to a common problem among shepherds.

"A little. And some signs of arthritis and calcification

of the spine. Don't get me wrong, she's a healthy dog, and loves her work."

"But you don't want to push her until she's hurting."

"I'm glad you understand."

"I do, which is why this is difficult to tell you. I have no puppies now. I wish I had."

"Ohhhh. I'd so hoped . . ."

The conversation lapsed into silence. Beth absently doodled on her notepad, not knowing what to say.

"I've just thought of something," Joanne exclaimed. "There's an excellent breeder of white shepherds in Winnipeg. Her name is Sharon Mann. In fact, she's got a litter now from her Seka and my Pancho."

"Do you think any are suitable?"

"I can't say, but I do know that Pancho gives every pup he sires great intelligence, drive, and willingness to learn. If any dog could sire search-and-rescue pups, it would be Pancho."

"Are there any males? Panda is an alpha bitch, and I don't think she'd welcome another female."

"You'll have to call Sharon. Let me give you her number, and tell her I sent you."

"Thanks, Joanne. Maybe I can finally find my dog."

"I have a *love* of a pup for you," Sharon Mann bubbled. "Great play drive, highly intelligent, particularly active retrieval skills, and a sweetheart to train."

"Male or female?"

"Male. He's four months old, and his name is Mansha's Sirius. Mansha for the kennel, of course, and Sirius for the dog star."

"He's named after a star?"

"That he is."

Beth had a hunch this was a match made in heaven. "I want him."

"He's yours."

Beth paced the freight hangar at the Minneapolis airport—up and down in a fever of impatience, waiting to see her new pup. Sharon had shipped him from Winnipeg to Minnesota, where Beth had flown to meet him and bring him home to Virginia.

"Here he is, lady," a freight handler called, pointing to a kennel he was pushing on a dolly.

Carefully Beth opened the crate. "Come, Siri."

A large, beautifully developed dog with a coat of ivory white stepped close to her and sniffed her hand. His eyes were the purest amber, and they locked on hers for an instant before he gave her hand a tentative swipe with his tongue.

"Good-looking dog, lady," the freight handler commented.

"Yes, he is, isn't he?"

Siri stretched, and those strange amber eyes of his almost twinkled at Beth. "I think this is the beginning of a beautiful friendship," she said, smiling at her new companion.

The Northwest Airlines jet was halted on the runway. And Beth was getting scared. The puppy was trapped in the cargo hold of the plane with the temperature climbing. Beth unbuckled her seat belt, and walked swiftly toward the cockpit.

A flight attendant blocked her path. "Please remain seated with your seat belt fastened."

"I have to see the captain."

"I'm afraid that's not possible. Is something wrong? Maybe I can help."

Beth grabbed her arm. "Tell the captain I have a puppy in the hold, and this heat could kill him."

"And your name is . . . ?"

"Beth Barkley. The pup is being trained for search-and-rescue work."

The flight attendant gave Beth a gracious, practiced smile. "I'll give him the message. Now if you'll kindly take your seat."

Beth swallowed her frustration and sat down. A few moments later, the static of the intercom buzzed. "This is the captain. I'm afraid we're experiencing further delays, and the tower informs me we will be sitting on the runway for at least another forty minutes. Sorry, folks. Would passenger Beth Barkley please get in touch with a flight attendant?"

Beth jumped from her seat and hurried toward the woman who had helped her before.

"Don't worry, Ms. Barkley. Come with me."

The attendant led her to the top of a flight of stairs that the captain requested be pushed up to the plane. The pilot stood at the bottom, directing the opening of the forward cargo doors himself. He glanced up at Beth. "You the lady with the pup?"

She nodded.

"Well, this'll cool things off in there. We'll keep the doors open until we get the word to move. Don't worry. I love dogs, too. Got a cocker spaniel at home. We'll make sure your pup's got some extra water, and he'll be fine."

"Thank you. I was so worried."

"Glad to help."

* * *

Sirius paced the backseat of Beth's car during the ride home from the airport, none the worse for his trip. Beth silently blessed the sympathetic captain, who might very well have saved Siri's life.

The pup watched everything that flew by him. Beth opened one window and he stuck his head out, enjoying the wind on his face in the mysterious manner of all dogs. Occasionally he pulled in his panting tongue and thrust his snout forward when something caught his eye.

Beth had thought it best that Panda meet the "new kid" at a neutral spot, rather than on home territory. A friend was scheduled to bring Panda to the school playground a few blocks from her house.

She cruised the parking lot until she spotted the two. She parked, clipped Siri's leash in place, and let him out to meet the queen of the roost.

Panda circled Siri, sniffing and nudging. Siri responded in an eager, puppy fashion, jostling the older dog, butting against her, leaping a few feet away, then planting his legs and daring her to chase him.

"Easy now, easy," Beth soothed.

Panda glanced at Beth, then Siri. She turned her back on the puppy and began to groom herself. *Well, at least she's not attacking him,* Beth thought.

"Come," she called, and both dogs headed for the car. Siri tried to push in ahead of Panda. Pan stepped back and glanced at her mistress. "Yes." Beth laughed. "He's coming with us."

Again, the older dog attempted to enter the car, but the youngster jostled her aside. Panda rounded on the pup, her teeth bared, a rumble erupting from her throat.

"Yip!" Siri cried, backing away.

Regally, the veteran turned and entered. Siri followed,

his tail tucked between his legs. The queen of the pack sprawled on the seat with an "all's right with the world" look on her face, leaving Siri a tiny spot, which he humbly took.

"Welcome home, Sirius." Beth laughed, and climbed aboard.

CHAPTER 9

LITTLE GIRL LOST

July 31, 1987, Richmond, Virginia

Eight-year-old Jo C. flicked her long, reddish-brown hair over her shoulders and curled her legs into a cross-legged squat, trying to get comfortable on the wooden dock that jutted into the lake behind her house. She dropped her baited hook in the water, sighed, and glanced around. Thick woods crowded the shoreline, broken every once in a while by the green expanse of lawn indicating a lakefront home or park.

It was a lovely setting, and a beautiful day. For that she was glad. But she was new to the neighborhood, and hadn't really made friends yet, so she was here alone.

"Any luck?"

Jo was startled by the friendly voice, and squinted up at the tall stranger with longish brown hair and a scruffy beard. She liked his smile. "No. Not a bite."

The man squatted beside her. "What you usin' for bait?"

"I have a worm I dug out of the dirt."

"I've fished in these parts before. I usually have luck with blood worms."

"Where do I get those?"

"Up at the 7-Eleven. You gotta buy 'em."

"I don't have any money."

The man absently threw a stone into the water. He touched Jo's arm and pointed across the lake. "See where the trees come right to the shore over there?"

The little girl nodded.

"That's where you can find bass. Sometimes a yellow perch. They're real tasty fish."

"Mom said if I caught anything, we'd have it for dinner."

"Did she? My mama used to do that. She sounds real nice, your mama."

"She is. I wish I could get her a fish."

The man cocked his head and looked at her as if considering. "Well, you know, I'm not doin' nothin'. What time you supposed to be home?"

"About 2:30."

"What do you say I drive you over there, and we try for a half hour? If we don't catch nothing, I'll take you home."

"That's real nice of you, mister."

"Nah. It'll be fun."

By 3:00, Jo's mother knew something was wrong. Her little girl was usually prompt, and she wasn't on the dock. "Maybe she's found a friend," the woman prayed, as she left the house to scour the neighborhood.

The 911 operator logged the call at 8:00 that evening. "I want to report my eight-year-old daughter as missing," Jo's father stated.

Ten minutes later, the police were knocking on their door.

* * *

Beth pulled up to the scene and let Panda out of the car just as Brooke Holt and her Rottweiler Buster hurried past.

"Hey, Beth," Brooke called. "Glad to see you."

"Hi. Same here."

Other handlers and dogs were present, as well as paramedics, emergency medical technicians, and rescue workers. There were at least five squad cars, as well as assorted ambulances and fire trucks. Lights whirled and changed colors in the night; reflecting off the lake, they made the neighborhood seem a macabre carnival. Helicopters beat the air, their spotlights illuminating great patches of trees for an instant before moving on.

Beth walked to Brooke. The rescue workers had been joined by a crowd of neighbors at least a hundred strong, who had volunteered to help the police.

"We got an eight-year-old girl gone missing. She was last seen fishing right off that dock," the sheriff bellowed. "We don't know if she's hurt, or maybe in the lake. . . ." The crowd groaned. "Or maybe she was snatched. We don't know."

"What do you mean, 'snatched'?" one of the neighbors asked.

"Possible abduction, ma'am," the officer answered.

The crowd caught their breath in shock.

"We're sending you neighbors into the woods. The dogs will stick to the lake."

Boats pulled to the dock as assignments were given. One of the dogs would do a water search, riding in the boat, trying to detect human scent drifting up through the water. If Jo was in the lake, the dog could smell her. Beth and Brooke were assigned to search the shoreline.

"Find 'em, Pan," Beth commanded. Her shepherd

stepped gingerly along the swampy lakefront, treacherous with tree roots and hidden vines. They were trailed by two medical techs. Occasionally, Beth could make out Brooke's light, and caught a glimpse of Buster prowling. Unlike Pan, Buster was as dark as the night; only the luminescent white cross on her shabrack showed the animal's location.

Powerful flashlights stabbed in and out of the darkness beneath the trees, and the night echoed with desperate cries from one hundred voices.

"Jo!"

"Jo, where are you?"

"Jo, can you hear me?"

The only answer came from the singing frogs, the whirring night insects, and the beating helicopter blades.

By 3:00 A.M., both Beth and Brooke had finished their sections and found no sign of Jo. Most of the neighbors had drifted back to the command center, reporting no luck. One comfort came from the fact that the dogs on the lake had found nothing either.

"We'll resume the search tomorrow, at oh-six-thirty," the incident commander stated. "This time, we concentrate on the woods."

Jo had been missing for fifteen hours.

Beth hadn't been able to sleep, thinking about the little girl and the search ahead of them. By 6:30, the field commander had maps of the area divided into grids, and had copied pictures of Jo. These were assigned to the volunteers, now two hundred strong.

Brooke and Beth, their dogs, and their tech partners

were assigned parallel grids—Brooke to the Cornerstone Church area, Beth to the lower swampy section.

"Good luck, Brooke," Beth called before they started. "If she's in your area, I know Buster will find her."

"Same with you," Brooke said. "Let's pray we do."

Conditions were easier for the search that morning. The sun was shining, there was a breeze, and the day promised not to be so hot that it would inhibit the dogs' abilities to detect human scent. It looked at least hopeful.

Jo had been missing for twenty-two hours.

The static from Beth's radio would stop every once in a while to emit voices reporting back to the command center. But there was nothing but empty news—and, stretched out before them, nothing but empty woods.

Suddenly, the radio cracked again. "This is Brooke Holt. Status 2. I repeat: Status 2. Over."

"Status 2" meant "found victim, need medical assistance."

"We're bringing her out."

"Yeah!" Beth yelled.

In the distance, she could hear cheering, as if crowds in a stadium were celebrating a touchdown. Brooke's words had been picked up at base.

"Panda," Beth called. *"Ven."* And away they ran, following the med tech angling to intercept Brooke and Buster. Status 2 was not the best news. It indicated problems, but how serious, they couldn't know.

They broke into a clearing and saw Brooke's med tech partner cradling an almost lifeless form in his arms. "She's bleeding. She's got wounds in the chest."

Beth could see a mass of tangled hair surrounding a face so chalk white every freckle stood out. Everywhere else the little girl was red-brown from blood—blood dripping down her neck, over her chest, sliding down her legs.

"Looks like puncture wounds . . . possibly a knife," the med tech said. "In the chest, neck. I see at least three, maybe more."

"Go, get her out of here," the second med tech urged, and the first man ran toward the waiting ambulance. Brooke and Beth sprinted after, their dogs close behind.

"You did it, Brooke," Beth cried, watching the ambulance speed up the street. "Good for you. Good, Buster. Good girl."

Brooke nodded. "I hope she makes it. That little girl is hurt awfully bad."

"Was she unconscious when you found her?"

"I'm not sure. Buster licked her face, and her eyes opened, but she didn't say a word. Poor baby. I'd like to get my hands on the scumbag who did this to her."

"If you hadn't found her, Brooke, she couldn't have lasted another night."

"What d'you mean if *I* hadn't found her? I was lucky to be assigned the sector where she was."

"I know that. But if you and Buster weren't so good, she might still be out there."

Brooke smiled, watching Buster play with her stick reward. "She's a good dog, isn't she?"

"Yeah. They all are."

Jo survived her hellish experience. She had been strangled, stabbed four times in the neck and chest, and left for dead by the "nice" stranger.

Showing remarkable courage throughout her ordeal, the eight-year-old was able to give the police a detailed description of her assailant. Two days later, they arrested a man who pleaded guilty to the assault on Jo. He is now serving three consecutive life sentences.

The entire team rejoiced in the success of their search. Many did not end so happily.

CHAPTER 10

LIFE OR DEATH

Two Months Later

Sugar Loaf Mountain, in the foothills of the Blue Ridge in northern Maryland, rounded softly into the azure sky, adorned in its seasonal best of crimsons and golds.

The day had been a scorcher, but a blessed chill descended with the sun's retreat. Beth and Marion Hardy leaned against Beth's Blazer, exhausted but triumphant.

"I think we gave them a show, Beth."

Beth glanced at the disappearing vans of the delegates from Partners of the Americas. "I think we gave them a great show, Marion."

Partners of the Americas was a government-sponsored international group that met in Washington three or four times a year. Sometimes they discussed trade, sometimes they exchanged medical knowledge. But this time, the group was investigating rescue techniques. All day, Beth and Pan, and Marion and Kerry, her black-and-tan shepherd, had demonstrated the astounding ability of their dogs. The two women had hidden members of the delegation all over the park, allowing their dogs to find them one by one. And find them Panda and Kerry did, no matter how the delegates tried to cover their tracks.

Never again would the Partners of the Americas doubt the skill of dogs to air-scent their way to victims. Leashed, ground-sniffing tracker dogs might need a piece of the victim's clothing for scent guidance and a fresh trail to follow; but Panda and Kerry, and dogs like them, needed no such tools. All they required was the breeze, and freedom to follow it.

Beth massaged her thigh muscles and stretched. It had been a grueling day. Even the intrepid Panda looked beat. She leaned against the side of the truck as if needing support. Beth knelt next to her, rubbing her gently. She could hear Pan's labored panting. "Are you all right, *perrita de mi corazón?*"

"Has she had enough water?" Marion questioned. "She might be dehydrated."

Beth shook her head. It was her cardinal rule that Panda be well watered, even if she herself had to go thirsty. "I know it's not dehydration."

"Is it the heat, do you think?" Marion asked, stooping next to the white shepherd.

"That could be it." Pan's deep, chocolate eyes turned to her mistress, a look of pure suffering in their depths. "*Mi amiga*, what's wrong?"

As if in answer, Panda swayed uncertainly and collapsed, unconscious. Beth caught the shepherd in her arms before she hit the ground. "Oh, my God! Help me, Marion. Help me get her into the truck."

Don't panic. If it had been anybody or any animal other than Pan, her practiced cool would have shifted to automatic. Now she had to force it.

Carefully, the women placed the limp shepherd into the truck, and Beth immediately began to dribble cool water along the length of her body. Within a few moments, Pan lifted her head, her tongue lolled into a more relaxed pant. Her eyes were no longer glazed.

"I think it must have been the heat," Marion said. "I'd get her home, let her play with Siri, and give her a light meal . . . and one for yourself while you're at it."

"As always, Marion, it's tough to argue with you. You're just too logical."

"It's a gift."

The next morning, Panda tried to walk toward her mistress. Slowly, the shepherd lifted one paw and placed it on the ground in a strange fashion as though not quite certain where her feet were. Then she paused, gathering strength again. Her whole body trembled with the effort. Another paw was lifted, and set down. Pause and tremble. Another paw placed gingerly as the dog strove to get to Beth. Even Siri backed away from her, his ears flattened, puzzled by the older dog's behavior.

"*Mi buen amiga.* I'm here. I'll come to you."

Beth knelt beside her, and took one of Panda's back paws into her hands. Gently, she turned it upside down, performing a common neurological test. If Panda's response was to stand on her toes, it meant her brain was not sending signals in a normal fashion. Panda stood tiptoe on all three of her remaining feet.

"Oh, no," Beth whispered.

Dr. Cockrill, Beth's friend and the best veterinarian she had ever known, moved his stethoscope to yet another part of Panda's chest. He listened intently to the animal's heart and lungs.

The doctor lifted his head, and tugged at his stethoscope until the tubes came out of his ears and rested on either side of his neck. His dark brown fingers ruffled Panda's light fur, a contrast that Beth focused on, waiting for his diagnosis.

Finally his sienna eyes sought hers. "Panda's a very sick dog. I'm afraid there's nothing I can do for her."

Before Beth could choke out a reply, he laid a hand reassuringly on her arm. "That doesn't mean nothing can be done. I don't have the facilities here. But there is a hospital in Potomac with specialists on staff and twenty-four-hour-a-day vet techs. If anyone can find out what's wrong with Pan, they can."

"What do you think it is?" Beth begged.

"I don't know. It's her lungs, but more than that I can't say yet. I do know she might die if she doesn't get help, and soon."

Beth watched Panda through a small, round window. The dog lay limp and apathetic inside an oxygen tent. For days, her shepherd had been poked and prodded, turned inside out, stuck with needles until Beth wondered if her *perrita* had any blood left in her gaunt body.

Panda was so helpless in her misery, so alone. The animal's ribs were outlined starkly, pushing through the skin, her stomach pinched because she'd lost so much weight.

Beth couldn't even touch her dog—offer her a loving caress. "I'm here, girl. I haven't deserted you." *Please don't die,* she added in her heart, because she couldn't say the words out loud.

"Ms. Barkley?"

A white-coated veterinarian stood by her side. "Yes?"

"Could you come with me? I think we know what's causing Panda's illness."

Finally. Beth entered a small, cramped office filled with pictures of cats and dogs, calendars advertising animal food, thank-you notes from grateful pet owners.

The doctor indicated a chair, and sat opposite her. "As you know, Panda's lungs are dreadfully scarred. We think it's a form of toxoplasmosis, but Panda has not responded to any of the antiviral drugs or the normal antibiotics we use to combat it."

"I know."

"Has Panda been out of the country recently?"

"Panda is a search-and-rescue dog."

The vet rifled through a manila file folder. "I see it here, in her records."

"Do you remember the earthquake in El Salvador last year?"

He nodded.

"We were part of the rescue team."

The doctor scratched behind his right ear with a pencil. "Did she inhale any dirt? Mouth any foreign substances? Possibly swallow any?"

Beth almost laughed. "Do you have any idea what earthquake damage is? Panda and I were on hills of rubble that used to be buildings searching for both the living and the dead. The question here should be 'where *didn't* she sniff dirt, where *didn't* she mouth foreign objects?' "

"So Panda didn't stay inside?"

"Hardly."

Again the man scratched thoughtfully with the eraser of his pencil. "That explains why she isn't responding."

"Could you fill me in, Doctor?"

"The bugs eating Panda's lungs are tropical, Ms. Barkley. We've got to change her course of treatment."

"Do you mean to tell me Panda's sick because of something she caught in El Salvador? A year ago?"

"Looks like it. It's toxoplasmosis, all right. It's simply a different form of the parasite than the one found in the States."

Beth was stunned. It wasn't fair. How could Panda be rewarded for all the good she had done with this illness that was eating her alive? "What will you do?"

"Now that we know it's tropical, I'm ordering new medications immediately. We'll do our best. I know she's strong, but honestly, she can't last much longer."

The doctor insisted that Beth stay at home. "It's like a patient in intensive care. It's best if they're not disturbed by visitors."

Beth understood—but it didn't comfort her any. Especially when her strength ebbed, and she allowed herself to think in terms of the worst. *Don't let her die alone. Please let me have the chance to say good-bye.*

Even Siri moped about the house. Beth tried to get him interested in a romp in the backyard between phone calls to the hospital but he wouldn't play. The pup sensed her depression.

She glanced at the clock. Wasn't it time to check on Pan again? Beth picked up the phone and requested to speak to the vet.

"Ms. Barkley?" This time the doctor sounded excited. "She's responding. Panda's finally responding. Her fever is down. Can you hear me? Ms. Barkley?"

Beth could hear him, all right—as clear as cathedral bells on Easter morning. Only she couldn't answer. She was crying too hard. She'd always read about tears of joy. It was the first time she'd ever experienced them.

Four weeks later, Panda trotted into the kitchen after a brief run around the backyard. Her weakness, her tiredness had lasted until only two days before.

But this morning, she bounced up as if the nightmare of the past weeks had been just that: a dream. She ate heartily, chased a robin that had not yet ventured south, batted around her favorite Frisbee, and nipped at Siri, letting him know she was once again the queen of the pack.

"What would I do without you, Pan?" Beth asked as the shepherd eased closer for a rub. "That's something I don't want to find out too soon."

CHAPTER 11

DISASTER—ARMENIA

Leninakan, December 7, 1988

A thick haze of diesel and sulfur fumes hung over Soviet Armenia's second-largest city, permeating the air with a sour thickness that not even winter's cold and snow could dissipate. People bustled about their mid-morning activities, irritated by the noxious fog that choked their once-pristine skies. But it was a legacy of Russian occupation they had learned to live with.

Another legacy of conquest was the relentlessly identical blocks of Soviet apartment buildings. They shadowed the centuries-old cathedral and the medieval squares like bullies; the beauty of the older buildings shamed the severe, ugly upstarts. These were relics of the time when the city had been named Alexanderapol, after Alexander the Great.

Inside, grandmothers cared for grandchildren whose parents had left for work. At the local college a teenage couple took advantage of the deserted, locked library to enjoy a lovers' tryst. In schools, children ignored the omnipresent face of Lenin, and furtively watched the clocks. Only four minutes until recess, and they would be free.

It was heard before it was felt—a roaring thunder that came, not from the skies, but from the earth. The stable, dependable ground shifted, then rolled in waves before it heaved upward in merciless violence. For an eternal ninety seconds, the land shuddered the city off its back as a dog would a flea. Three minutes passed quietly; then it shook again. In those few minutes, Leninakan was reduced to rubble. Tens of thousands were trapped in their homes, offices, and schools; thousands were dead or dying. All the public clocks were frozen at one time, as if eternity had begun at 11:41 A.M.

Virginia, December 8, 10:11 A.M.

Beth closed the front door behind her just as the telephone rang. "Darn." Should she ignore it? No, she couldn't resist its incessant demands. She fumbled with her keys, flung open the door, and made a flying grab for the receiver.

"Beth? It's Ralph Wilfong. Consider this your 'heads up' from OFDA. We're placing dog teams and overhead on alert. If needed, can you and Panda go?"

"Where?"

"The Soviet Union. Armenia."

"I have to call my boss at AT&T. He's usually sympathetic. If he'll give me a leave of absence, I can come."

Yerevan, December 11, 5:15 A.M.

The Air America 727 buzzed the airport. This was the third time the pilot had circled, frustrated by planes parked at chaotic angles on the one runway.

"Tower tells me relief supplies are coming in," the pilot announced. "It's a real mess down there. But not to worry. We'll have you good people on the ground as soon as we can."

Relief supplies. Beth remembered the spokesman for the State Department rattling off the statistics during their briefing back home. One hundred million dollars in aid from seventy-three countries, including two thousand rescue workers.

Inching into view below them was a nuclear power plant. Beth studied the immense smoke stacks and the squat, ugly bunkers powdered with grayish-black, polluted snow. She wondered what damage the earthquake had inflicted on the facility. Were they flying into another Chernobyl?

The jet banked steeply and Beth sucked in her breath. She heard the same reactions from other members of the team, but the dogs were handling it much better than their persons.

Carol and Steve McConaughy's magnificent Newfoundlands, Ebony and Shasta, sprawled next to them, eyes closed. Brooke Holt soothed Buster, the Rottweiler who'd found the kidnapped girl in Virginia the year before. The mass of golden fur reclining across Pat Yessel's lap was her retriever Rubble. Caroline Hebard's Aly sat upright, attentive. A second black-and-tan, Grief, belonged to Ed Johnson, a strapping six feet six inches of a man. And Tim and Penny Sullivan, veterans from New Jersey, brought the third and fourth black and tan shepherds.

Beth turned to catch a glimpse of the rest of the strike squad. Joaquin del Cueto, a Metro-Dade firefighter and paramedic, had enjoyed every hospitality the attendants had directed his way during the flight. Now he leaned back, snoring like a well-fed emperor. *Nerves of steel.* Beth had observed his unflappable cool in El Salvador, and was delighted to work with him again.

Scattered about the jet were various members of the State Department, emergency physicians, members of relief groups. They numbered forty-two in all—the largest humanitarian aid effort the United States had sent to the Soviet Union since World War II.

But Beth wondered about volunteer civilians in the group. Too many of them had invaded the duty-free shops at Shannon Airport in Ireland to buy sweaters, because they'd not thought to bring warm clothes. A prime example of this senselessness could be seen a few rows up. Sticking into the aisle were two sockless feet, clad in open-heel clogs. The feet belonged to a doctor from California. By what logic the man had concluded that clogs were the footwear of choice for winter in Armenia, Beth couldn't begin to guess. What else had he packed? Hawaiian shirts?

Another swing of the jet brought Beth's stomach into her throat and her thoughts to the dangers ahead. "I can't worry about those guys, Pan," she whispered to the dog whose deep eyes always seemed to understand. "We're finally in Armenia, and we can't even land the plane!"

She spoke from frustration. The "hurry up and wait" mentality was getting to her. It had been four days since the earthquake, three days since Ralph Wilfong's initial "heads up" call. "No go," he told her when he phoned later that day. "We're on," he said twelve hours later. The team was flown from Dulles to New York, then back to Dulles before they finally headed overseas.

The organizing, shuffling around, and waiting made

her crazy. The window of survival, twenty-four to thirty-six hours after a disaster, had slammed shut, and there was not a thing she could do about it.

Panda remained calm, her pink tongue lolling, every now and then flicking the tip of her pink nose. "I wish I had your patience, *mi perrita*."

Beth gripped the armrest of her seat as the plane made a fifth circle. The jet headed toward the runway, rapidly losing altitude. "Yes! Pan, I think we're going to see some action at last."

HURRY UP AND WAIT . . . AGAIN

"Please let the zipper hold," Beth muttered as her enormous purple duffle, stuffed to the gills, hit the tarmac.

The rescue workers stood in line at the baggage compartment and bumped out their equipment. The team didn't hear the truck that pulled up behind them. Nobody got out. The Russian soldiers who'd greeted them moments before made no move to help.

"We're strong, right, Beth?" Carol McConaughy laughed. "We got to haul it here. We get to pack it on a truck."

"Let's move, people," their team leader directed.

"*Sientate,* Panda," Beth commanded, and Pan sat, alert, watching Beth's every move.

From nowhere a knot of men appeared beside them. Dark, intelligent eyes stared out from strong features surmounted by ice-tipped hats. One of the group rushed to Beth as she dragged her duffle. A flash of tobacco-stained teeth accompanied the smile of concern. He tugged gently on her bag.

"No, no," Beth said, returning his smile. "I can do it."

The man nodded, said something in a language that was certainly not Russian, and turned to haul a crate to the truck. *He's Armenian,* Beth thought. *They've come to help us.*

Another Armenian approached Carol in the same polite manner, offering to carry her burdens. But Carol's reaction was the same as Beth's. Finally, the men realized that the American women pulled their own weight, and soon they were working side by side with the strike team, both men and women.

"Thank you. Thank you," one of them kept repeating.

"This is refreshing," Beth remarked to Joaquin del Cueto. "Half the time, I thought those *capitalinos* were going to stone us. So far, these guys are grateful we came."

"Makes it nice. Now, if we'd get going, I'd be real happy."

3:00 P.M.

"Can't we get going?" Joaquin groaned. "It's been ten hours, and all we've done is ride around this airport."

"We have to arrange transportation and make sure our visas are valid."

This had been the State Department dirge all day. Beth didn't bother to look at the person chanting it now.

A wave of Turkish tobacco smoke wafted into her face and a fit of coughing left her in spasms.

"You okay?" Brooke Holt asked.

Beth wiped at her streaming eyes. "Yeah."

"I swear I don't know what's worse," Brooke sighed, glancing around the smoke-filled expanse, "the air inside the terminal, or the air outside the terminal."

"I'm opting for outside," Beth choked. "Want to come?"

"Too cold for me, thanks."

"*Aquí,* Pan." She smacked her leg, and pushed into the caustic air outside. The pollution hung thick, gray, and heavy, as if she were breathing inside a chimney flue. *Brooke's right,* she thought. *This is just as bad.*

A Soviet jet taxied toward the terminal, then stopped. Shuffling, silent men, women, and children streamed out of the plane. Some were dressed in scant bits and pieces, as if they'd pulled their clothes from rag bags. They shivered in the raw air. Their blue lips and gloveless, red fingers betrayed their misery as much as the resignation in their eyes. The U.S. team had been witnesses to the familiar sight all day, angry at their own helplessness.

A long articulated bus with an accordion midsection clattered toward the terminal, blocking Beth's view of the refugees. It screeched to a halt, smothering her with a dense cloud of fumes. Julia Taft of the State Department hopped out, spotted her, and smiled. She waved behind her at the bus. "It's ours. We're going to Leninakan."

"Leninakan? You mean it?"

"As soon as we get everybody packed up, we're out of here."

The team managed to squeeze in everything, including boxes and boxes of one-gallon water jugs, but still the bus idled. Some of the group huddled inside, driven by their craving for warmth. Others milled around a grassy area under the shelter of one sad, bare tree.

"What's up?" Caroline asked Beth. "Why aren't we leaving?"

"Beats me."

"I'm going to find out." She headed toward Julia Taft.

In the distance, Beth could see the two peaks of Mount Ararat. Under the snow, legend tells, the great ark of Noah rests. When the winter is mild, some have claimed to have seen the ark entombed in ice.

"A mild winter? Right," she said to the shepherd. Beth noticed she talked a lot to Pan lately—ever since her partner's bout with toxoplasmosis. Maybe she was being overprotective. Panda appeared in perfect health, just like her old self. Still, Beth worried about her best friend. She snuggled the dog closer, protecting her from the blasts of frigid air nipping and swirling around them. "I'm taking Panda inside if we don't leave soon," she said to Ralph. He shrugged and looked as disgusted as she felt.

"We'll leave in just a minute." Julia Taft spoke breathlessly. Her cheeks glowed like those of a girl going to her first dance. "See that?"

All Beth could see were three old helicopters, circa 1950, and two shiny new ones. "What?"

"Didn't you hear? Gorbachev will be here any minute. He's going to inspect the damage."

"That's why we're sitting?"

She got no answer, and realized all eyes were focused behind her. She turned in time to watch a long limousine, surrounded by several black Citroens, sprinting toward them. Tiny red flags fluttered on either side of the limo's hood.

"There he is," someone shouted.

Beth could barely make out the man hustled from the

bowels of the limo into the waiting state-of-the-art copter. The blades revved and beat the air. Beth hunched her shoulders against the wind, and covered Panda's ears with her hands. The craft hovered, tilted, and traveled along the ground in their direction, slowly gaining speed but no altitude.

"Look out!" someone yelled. "It's heading right for us."

"Get down!" Beth screamed. She dove on top of Panda.

The helicopter ascended, its blades ripping off the branches of the tree directly above them. Splinters, twigs, dirt, and minced leaves showered down on them.

"Welcome to Armenia." Beth was shaking as she stood up and dusted off Panda.

5:30 P.M.

The terrain between Yerevan and Leninakan began as stretches of plains between hills that rose into snow-covered mountains.

The bus topped a rise, and although she should have known better after two hours careening through the Armenian countryside on roads crowded with frantic drivers, Beth looked through the windshield. Heading straight for them, all jammed into the same lane, were no less than three cars.

Beth pulled Panda between her legs and laughed from pent-up nerves, frustration, and terror. She squeezed her eyes tight, and braced for the inevitable head-on collision she knew was going to kill them all before they even got within sight of Leninakan.

Nothing. She looked again. The cars had scattered—but now a dirty yellow truck pitched toward them, the crosshairs of its headlights beamed straight into Beth's face. Then it, too, miraculously avoided smashing into them.

"I'm going to have a heart attack," someone groused.

Beth had never experienced such a thrill ride as the road to Leninakan. On a meager four-lane road with iffy shoulders, the Armenian drivers created seven lanes of traffic—no guarantee that they were all headed in the same direction. Hooting, honking, and wild gestures stirred up the chaos. Pan finally had enough, and rested her head in her mistress's lap, one paw draped across her knees.

"Good idea," Beth commented, and decided to try to imitate her dog's calm. She watched the countryside bump past and endeavored to be charmed. Grapevines were everywhere. The humblest cottage had its arbor attached.

"See that building?" The doctor from California pointed. "That's where they make Armenian cognac. The best in the world."

"Got any handy?" Beth asked.

The bus rolled into the afternoon. The ride offered no escape from the scenes of destruction. One particular sight stopped all conversation: A few miles outside the city, the smoking white tail of a Soviet jet jutted out at a crazy angle from a mountainside. Beth had heard of this accident while waiting in Yerevan, but had never seen anything like it. The plane had crashed with such force it had fashioned a stark halo of charred, burned debris around itself. No person was near the site; only wheel tracks in the snow showed any attempt at recovery efforts.

This was the domino effect of disaster. The plane had been carrying Russian rescue workers—sixty-nine servicemen and nine crew members. All were killed.

. Leninakan rose from the chill face of the plain. The city started abruptly with a magnificent, modern church still standing, a defiant reminder that this was a practicing, and prosperous, Christian country.

"I like these people already, Pan," Beth whispered. "I'm glad we came."

Twenty nine-story apartment houses marked the edge of town. Two-thirds were collapsed; the others were so heavily damaged, they were dangerous and empty. Burned seams of glowing crimson veined through the rubble. Black soot sparked by flames belched into the darkening sky. The crumpled buildings painted eerie silhouettes against the unnatural light. The broken windows of one smashed store spilled its Christmas decorations onto the street, casting strangely festive greens, golds, and reds on the dirty snow.

Everyone fell silent.

The bus pushed deeper into the chaos and now the rescue workers were faced with the citizens of Leninakan. Crowds of men and women, strange, blank looks stamped on their handsome faces, scurried in between masses of overcoated Soviet soldiers—a population in shock and under siege.

Some tried to board the bus as it stalled at an intersection, hoping it was going somewhere, anywhere, away from here. Others lugged furniture and clothing from unstable buildings, trying to save what scraps of their lives they could. Color-coded coffins of various sizes were piled on sidewalks, their dead waiting to be claimed by relatives. An Armenian man trudged by, unnaturally bowed by the tiny coffin balanced on one shoulder.

A low, strange "grrwoof" rumbled from Panda's throat. "Ssshhh, Pan," Beth whispered, shocked by her first sight of this soon-to-be-familiar scene.

"Spitak was the hardest-hit area. Smack on the epicenter. It was wiped out," Julia Taft said.

Harder hit than this? How could that be?

This ancient city must surely have been unrecognizable to these people who had survived the Apocalypse. The ragged remnants of buildings looked like stage sets, their outside walls sheared off to reveal intimate glimpses into the ruin of people's lives. Every precious heirloom—a lost daughter's hair ribbons, a Persian rug handed down from grandmother to mother, photos of cherished faces—was trampled underfoot or piled on rubble mountains.

"Eighty percent of the population in Leninakan is homeless," Julia Taft continued. "There are no hospitals, no utilities, no communications. Nothing. The count so far is more than one hundred thousand casualties, over fifty-five thousand dead." She recited the data as if it were imprinted on her brain.

Although Beth had heard the statistics earlier, the enormity of the disaster had been hard to comprehend until she'd seen Leninakan for herself. They must begin searching soon.

Finally, the bus circumnavigated the confusion of the town square and stopped. "I'm going to find the mayor," Julia announced. "The rest of you stay here. We don't have permission for you to roam around."

"You just want us to sit?" Beth asked.

"I think we could get out and do some good right now, right here," Caroline added in a measured tone.

"I'm afraid that's not possible," Julia stated. "We'll be back as soon as we can. Please just sit tight."

Beth's hands fisted impatiently. "I've got to get out of this bus. Panda has to be able to walk around, and so do I."

"I'm with you," Ralph Wilfong answered.

So was every other member of the rescue team.

But it was 9:00 P.M. before the Americans were allowed to start searching. They found no survivors that first night.

IMPRESSIONS

Day Two: December 12, 5:30 A.M.

Snow had fallen inside the massive Russian tent. Beth groaned and looked for leaks until she realized it was the moisture from the animals and humans that had condensed and frozen into a miraculous minisnowfall.

Panda tried to turn in the sleeping bag she shared with her mistress, but there was no room. They had four blankets doubled under them, and four blankets on top, yet neither had been able to get warm in their restless, chilly two and a half hours of sleep.

Beth struggled up and pulled on every warm piece of clothing she had brought. Her long, blond hair, pulled tight into a functional French braid, was itching. She knew she smelled. She hadn't bathed for, what, three days now? Nor had she changed her clothes. She couldn't even wash her hands or face. Water was too precious for that. And she was cold—so unrelentingly cold.

Panda burst free of the sleeping bag, sighing and stretching, scratching and whining. "All right, *perrita de mi corazón*, we'll go out."

Their water had frozen during the night. Beth dragged a cookstove outside and worried a flame to life.

"Beth, would you hold this for me?" She turned just in time to catch the blanket Pat Yessel tossed in her direction.

"Oh, going to the powder room, are we?"

Pat grinned sheepishly. "Same place as last night?"

The two women headed to their alfresco bathroom at the back of the tent. Beth did a quick reconnoiter and held up the blanket. "Okay, all clear."

Pat ducked behind its flimsy privacy, and Beth contemplated her boots.

"Ooooh . . . ," sounded from behind the blanket.

Beth had to laugh.

"I can hear you," Pat complained. "You wait, it's your turn next."

"Well, hurry up or my bladder will burst."

The cookstove was doing its job. Beth's pot was simmering by the time the handlers got back to the front of the tent. Carol McConaughy peered out of the flap. "Beth, Shasta's in trouble. Steve said it's the beginnings of hypothermia."

"Coming." She carried the warm water inside and pushed her way through the group of people surrounding the Newfoundland. Steve and Carol had covered Shasta with their sleeping bags and were massaging her legs and paws. "Get this down her."

"Thanks," Carol said, taking the warm water from Beth.

The couple had caught Shasta in time; Beth could go

back and heat Panda's water. "She'll be all right." Beth tried to sound reassuring as she left.

Beth hunched on her heels, watching the ice melt slowly as little bubbles formed at the bottom of the pot. The eastern sky lightened into a dull gray. This day melded into the last, a mélange of bleak, drab, and endless time without sun. There was a sense of no color, of stepping back into the past, of unreality.

"Miss . . . *bitte*?"

The heavily accented voice startled her. Beth stared into the haggard face of a woman whose eyes were livid with suffering. The Armenian swept an arm toward the wreckage of an apartment building. "My . . . um . . . *haus . . . helfen, bitte*." Beth understood the broken German with which the woman was attempting to communicate, but before she could answer, a weary male voice spoke.

"Sorry, lady. Not yet. We'll come as soon as we can," Bill Dotson said, as he stumbled from the tent.

The woman turned away as if expecting this response. Tears overflowed and dripped freely down her cheeks. She didn't bother to dash them away.

"Wait." Beth ran into the tent and grabbed one of her blankets, then hurried back to the Armenian. "Here. At least I can give you this."

The woman buried her face in its comfort for a silent moment. *"Danke."*

A drift of other figures were heading toward the Americans. More displaced people begging for help. They approached other members of the team, who in turn handed out their own precious blankets and tarps. Beth reluctantly went back to preparing breakfast.

Ralph Wilfong bent over the cooking stove. "Smells

decent," he said. "Then again, after twenty-four hours without food, I'll eat anything." He watched Beth stir the instant oatmeal for the humans, then the dog food—Alpo puppy chow mixed with Alpo canned food. "Glad you're using two spoons."

"When are we going to start, Ralph?"

"Your guess is as good as mine. They're moving us again."

"What? When?"

"Well, let's see. They said at 0630. Almost that now. If they're true to form, I think that buys us another five hours."

"Any objection if, after I get Panda fed, we head there?" Beth jerked her thumb at the Armenian woman's *haus*.

"Me? Object? Give everyone a bowl of oatmeal, then let's go."

Panda snorted to clear her receptors clogged by smoke and exhaust fumes. She moved cautiously over the reeking ruins of the apartment building, the shifting debris cascading from under her feet at each step. Beth followed closely to make sure her partner didn't step on a hot spot and burn her delicate pads.

The U.S. team soon discovered that the Soviet builders had not cared much for quality. They'd used a local rock—the porous, volcanic tuff—and cheated on the amount and quality of the concrete.

Standards for height and seismic restrictions had been ignored, too, so the buildings never had a chance to with-stand an earthquake that had measured 6.9 on the Richter scale; they had simply crumbled to dust. This meant there were few voids, other than stairwells or elevator

shafts, in which people could survive. The only compen-
sation for the team's difficult, dirty, dangerous work that
morning was that it was warmer in the belly of the
building than on top of it.

Yet Beth wondered if maybe someone had found that
poor woman's family. Underneath one of those orange
markers might be a son or daughter. Maybe tomorrow,
after the bodies had been removed, the Armenian woman
would find her family in coffins stacked on a curb. As
terrible as this seemed, it was better than nothing.

Afternoon

Joaquin del Cueto and Raoul Chavez from Metro-
Dade hailed their compatriots. "We rounded up some
transportation," Joaquin called.

"Great." Beth sighed. The team had been working spo-
radically in downtown Leninakan, but their bus had left
them to take their equipment to the new campsite. None
of the rescue workers were feeling very comfortable
separated from their supplies. And they'd given up on
finding anyone alive.

Beth called Panda, who was reclining on a thick piece of
wool. The workers at a nearby textile factory had brought
the fabric to the dogs to help keep them warm while the
team searched for the remains of friends and family.

"Did you get a van?" Beth asked Joaquin.

"Ah . . ." Joaquin hesitated. "You'll see. Follow me."

The only empty vehicle in the square was a massive
dump truck, the kind used in quarries. Joaquin led them
straight to it.

The back of the truck towered over Beth's head. The

bed itself was six feet off the ground. "You can't mean it," she said. "How on earth can any of us, let alone the dogs, haul ourselves into that thing?"

"Yeah, I had to cut a deal to get it, too," the Metro-Dade man answered.

"I don't know if I want to hear this. You better let us in on it."

"The driver will take you to your new camp at the airport if you'll search a factory and a college where the guy—"

"Let me guess. He's got some relatives he wants us to find." This was a familiar scenario when rescue workers had to bum rides from the local people.

"You got it."

Joaquin signaled the driver to back up to a decorative fountain and let down the gate. The strike team threw their packs into the truck. The first person climbed the fountain and crawled aboard.

Beth found a foothold on one satyr's prominent marble unmentionable and grabbed the breast of a nymph for support before she could hoist herself onto the bed. Other team members fountain-climbed in, sliding across the icy metal floor. Finally, Joaquin and Raoul lifted the dogs into the arms of their handlers.

Panda's back legs flailed in the air until she felt the solid floor under her. *"Aquí, perra,"* Beth murmured, spreading the runner of wool for them to sit on. The truck lurched to a start, and nearly everyone flipped heels over head.

"Great job, Joaquin," someone called as the dump truck jounced them around like pebbles on a plate. "Next time, why not a cement mixer?"

"Better'n walking," Joaquin answered good-naturedly. Beth wasn't too sure she'd bet the baby on that statement.

Beth followed Panda to the second floor of the destroyed college. The area over the central hallway had collapsed downward in one killing slab.

The white shepherd picked her way along. She whined and touched her nose to the floor, moved no more than an inch or two before she alerted again. This continued— one extended dead alert the whole length of the corridor. Under the porous chunk of rock the school was thick with corpses. Here and there a foot, an arm, an upper torso protruded. Beth left the area and slid after Panda onto the floor below, landing on her hip.

"You all right?" Joaquin called. He was her spotter.

"Yeah," she answered. "Ouch," she grumbled to herself, rubbing her side. She'd hit the same hip when she'd jumped from the dump truck, and from the feel of it, she'd bruised it pretty badly. This injury was going to give her trouble, especially in this frigid, wet city.

Beth brought out her flashlight. Two of the walls were still intact. Her slender beam played over fallen shelves and jumbled piles of ripped books. This had been a library.

She crawled after Panda, negotiating the ruins. Suddenly, the dog stopped, her pink nose tilted upward, her nostrils pulling in something.

"¿Donde está, Pan? Where is it?"

The shepherd scratched at a shelf blocking her way. A leather-bound tome fell to the floor, and Panda sidestepped, then nosed the volume aside. There was no enthusiasm, no eagerness in her alert.

Beth wormed under the shelf, and spied something

hidden behind an overturned table. She moved closer, and her invading light exposed a sad tableau. Entwined together, two young lovers had been caught by death in a last caress.

Beth lowered her eyes. It seemed obscene that she'd disturbed the peace of their eternal embrace. She stayed motionless, her head bowed, then marked the spot and crawled away. The lover's tryst was no longer secret.

The partners finished the room, finding no one else, and climbed back into the bleak, cloud-covered day.

Joulie, a young Armenian-American girl who had joined the team earlier that day as their interpreter, was waiting for Beth as she hit the surface.

"How's it going, Joulie?"

"I've talked to the people here."

Beth glanced at the men and women waiting for word of their children, sister, brother, or lover, and she didn't envy Joulie her job. "I'm sorry. That must have been rough."

"It was terrible. But I learned something. The students were on break when the quake struck, and most were in the hall."

That explained the corridor of death Panda had discovered. "What about the library?"

"No, nobody in there. The place was closed and locked at the time."

"You'd better tell them otherwise. They'll want to remove the bodies before they plow the building under."

Word of the couple in the library spread through the crowd. The boy and girl were easily identified, and their names whispered from one person to the next. It made death infinitely more personal to Beth, and infinitely more painful.

* * *

Snow was falling again. It clung to the coats of the dogs, and to the hats and gloves of the handlers.

"Is it ever going to end?" Beth rasped. Her hip throbbed, her throat was raw from the fumes, her head ached from lack of sleep.

She stretched and stood on tiptoe on the truck bed and tried to peer over the massive sides to see where they were going. All the jammed roads looked alike. She sat down.

She didn't like this battle-scarred transport. It reminded her of something out of *Star Wars*. Besides, Joulie had confided that before Joaquin had commandeered it, the vehicle had been used to haul the dead.

They lurched to a stop. At first Beth assumed it was traffic; then the engine cut off.

"I think we're here," Ralph said. "This must be our new camp."

The rescue workers groaned, rose to their feet, and crowded toward the tailgate. With a shrill shriek, the metal wall crashed open. The team surged forward, staring at the sight before them. Gradually, smiles replaced astonishment. Then came applause.

High on a pole, lit by a powerful wedge of light, the Stars and Stripes streamed and whipped against the night sky. Beth cheered with her mates. The American flag on Soviet soil!

In their enclave, other team sites had been set up. There was the Canadian maple leaf, and beside that, the Union Jack.

Familiar faces materialized out of the dark, Doug Jewett and Jimmy Arias from Metro-Dade among them. Doug was once again in charge of the men from Miami.

"Welcome to the Leninakan Hilton. It ain't the five-star Presidente, but it's home," he remarked as he reached to lift Panda to the ground. "I think I preferred the monsoons in El Salvador to the snow here. What d'ya think, Beth? I see you still got that worthless mutt of yours." Doug grinned and rubbed Panda until she writhed with delight.

"Yep. I'm sure you told everyone that our dogs aren't worth a snap of your fingers."

"Who, me?" he asked innocently.

Doug loved to bad-mouth the dog team. But Beth had seen in El Salvador that if Pan wasn't by her side, the shepherd was next to Doug, being petted and fussed over. "Yes, you. But I notice you call us quick enough when there's trouble."

"Beth, you're always trouble."

"And I always will be."

The two laughed, and joined the rest of the team.

Beth surveyed her surroundings. There were several huge piles covered by OFDA tarps; fifteen blue and white summer-weight tents; a concrete aqueduct that separated them from the road and the airport; and— miracle of miracles—their bus with all their gear intact.

"Hey," one of the firefighters yelled. "I'm hungry. Who's ordering the pizza?"

"Domino's delivers to Armenia," someone chimed back.

The image of the little Domino's delivery car dodging over the mountainous roads to Leninakan was infectious. Everyone roared.

"Let's get to work, people," Bill Dotson called.

Beth bent over the steel box the Metro-Dade men had set up as a permanent heater/stove. The wood fire threw inadequate heat, but it was the only heat.

She reached up to her itching head and gave it a luxurious scratch with both hands. Four days without bathing. *This, too, shall pass.*

She felt a tap on her shoulder, and turned. A Fairfax County firefighter stood behind her. "Aren't you Beth Barkley?"

Beth nodded, and looked closer at the man. Why was he so familiar?

"Don't you know me? I'm Butch Sisler."

"Butch?" All Beth could do was stare. Butch Sisler. Talk about a blast from the past. The two had gone from second to twelfth grade together, but hadn't seen each other since high school. Butch had married one of her schoolmates, and Beth remembered the wicked crush she'd had on the boy in fifth grade.

"Butch Sisler?"

"In the flesh. Can you believe it? How many years has it been—and we run into each other in *Armenia*? It takes coming halfway around the world and a major disaster to get us together. What's wrong with this picture?"

A lot, but Beth didn't care. She was too delighted to see her old buddy. "Butch Sisler," she repeated.

"Your conversation hasn't improved any," Butch laughed.

Beth grinned. "Butch Sisler," she said again. "How in the world are you doing?"

When Beth and Panda turned in it was late, yet the tent was so freezing she could only doze. Every fifteen minutes a Soviet jet roared overhead, and Panda would startle. "Shhh," Beth soothed. "Things will be better tomorrow." It was the first time she had lied to her dog.

"IS GOD AGAINST US, TOO?"

Day Three: December 13

Two firefighters from Fairfax County, Virginia, cast their lights into the gloom of a ruined building in Leninakan. "That doesn't look too good."

"Actually, it looks great," Beth commented. "See those supports? It's sturdy, and there'll be large hollows behind them with enough air that somebody might still be alive."

"Our people found some living yesterday."

Beth had heard about the grandmother, sheltered by a fallen refrigerator. Her two granddaughters had not been so lucky. They had died in their grandmother's arms, clinging so closely their bodies had made deep imprints into hers.

And everyone marveled at the fourteen-year-old girl who'd survived six days, her cries so feeble the Czech rescue workers thought they heard a kitten mewing.

"I'm going in," Beth said. She sat at the edge of the breadth of parquet that dipped into the darkness, gathered Pan into her lap, and shoved off. The surface was slick and her ride fast and scary. She skidded to the floor with a loud thump.

"Everything okay?" one of the firefighters called.

"Fine." *Except for my hip,* Beth thought, easing her weight off the offending joint.

Panda was already searching. She bounded a few feet away and scratched wildly. She circled back to Beth, then pranced around, leading her back.

Someone was alive. Beth fell to her knees. "Hello. Can

you hear me?" she called. Silence. She waved to her spotter. "Pan's giving a 'live' alert."

"Are you sure?"

"Yes! Yes! Tell Joulie to get some help here."

The second Fairfax man hurtled down the parquet slide and landed beside her. "See?" Beth said and pointed to Pan. The shepherd dug furiously in front of them.

The firefighter shrugged. The dog's animation meant nothing to him. One by one, six solid Armenian men slid alongside the Americans. Their leader tapped Beth on the shoulder and pointed up toward the opening. His message was clear, if unspoken. *You've done your job; let us do ours.*

Beth nodded. "We've got to go."

"You mean, we can't watch?" the firefighter asked.

"No. That's one of our big frustrations. We're the first in, and the first out, and it's rare somebody remembers to let us know if we were right."

"That bites."

"Can't argue with you there."

Joulie helped Beth water the white shepherd, who panted on the runner of factory wool Beth now carried everywhere.

"Panda's worn out," Joulie said, patting the dog.

"Too much death. By the time we go home, she'll be comatose."

"Hey, Beth," Joaquin joked as he passed. "Are you ordering the pizza tonight, or should I?"

"Your turn."

"Pizza?" Joulie asked.

"Yeah. The big joke at camp is that one of these nights, Domino's is going to deliver."

"So at least you're having a little fun."

Beth looked thoughtfully at the girl. Fun. It wasn't a word she'd use to describe what they were going through. "A laugh every now and then keeps us sane."

"I wish I could laugh."

Beth put a reassuring arm around Joulie's slender shoulders. The girl worried her. She was one of the lone intermediaries for the Americans, most of whom couldn't even decipher the alphabet of this exotic land.

How many times had Beth seen Joulie swallowed in a breaking crest of people, pulled apart by its undertow. The girl would jerk free, her face drained of color. The message was always the same. "This woman (man) heard her daughter (son, brother, mother) inside that building," she'd interpret. "If you could bring the dogs, they'll find them."

The team answered her proxied requests, although for the most part, they knew them to be the lies or hopes of the distraught. Joulie was bent under the emotional weight of it all, and Beth could only offer sympathy. The young student would have to learn to don armor herself.

A handsome woman approached. She kissed Beth on both cheeks, pressed a small jar into her hand, and left. It was filled with pimientos stuffed with celeriac in oil and garlic. "Thank you," she called after the woman, who waved and nodded.

"Where do they find the strength to be so generous?" Joulie asked. "They're starving."

"These are your people. Their courage will see them through this, and so will yours."

An elderly man tapped Joulie's arm and questioned with low, desolate words.

"He asks if you know from news abroad if this was a natural disaster or man-made. There are rumors that the Soviets caused a nuclear explosion."

Beth looked into rheumy, red eyes. "Seismologists around the world recorded this earthquake."

Joulie translated. The man was silent for a moment. When he spoke, his voice sounded like ice. He stalked away.

The interpreter covered her face, and leaned against Beth.

"What did he say to make you cry, Joulie?" Beth demanded.

"He asked, 'Is God against us, too, then?' "

His simple words carried the weight of centuries, the tears of affliction his people had wept throughout the ages—tears of such bitterness that they burned through even Beth's hard shell.

Both Americans cried, clinging to each other. An Armenian woman wrapped her arms around them, and rocked them gently. Who she was, where she'd come from—such considerations seemed trivial. Her simple gesture of comfort was enough.

At camp that night, Beth clung to the hope that someone had been pulled from the rubble where Panda had alerted that morning. No word had been sent. She would probably never know. She put her arms around her *perrita* and closed her eyes, but sleep was a long time coming.

A TERRIBLE MEASURE OF SUCCESS

Day Four: December 14, the nearby town of Kirkovan

"Ralph, you can't spot for both Carol and for me. That's dangerous, and I won't have it," Beth yelled at the startled spotter.

"Ooookay, I'll see what I can do."

"I'm sorry. I didn't mean to take it out on you."

"Good thing I'm a patient sort." Ralph smiled, and pulled out his radio.

Beth fought to keep her temper in check. This factory had produced the faulty concrete used in Leninakan's apartment buildings. But the manager, who spoke English, whispered bitterly to her that the people who were responsible for the poor quality of the concrete were not the people who had died here.

"I'll spot for you, Beth, if you don't bite my head off," Joaquin offered.

"Or you can take me," his buddy added. "But . . . be gentle."

"I promise," Beth said. "I didn't mean to lose it on Ralph. Anyway, Panda keeps wanting to go to the right, but your gang said it's not safe. What do you think?"

Joaquin pressed his lips to his radio. "Panda wants to check things on the right side. Can we? Over."

"As long as you're with her. Over."

"Let's go," Joaquin said.

Panda disappeared into the shadows ahead. Beth, Joaquin, and the second firefighter followed. Several bodies were piled together, blocking their path. Even in the cold, the smell of death was apparent.

"My God," Joaquin's buddy exclaimed.

Beth didn't look back. She climbed over the frozen remains and methodically checked the wing. It took Panda and her less than fifteen minutes. "We're done."

"How do we get out?" the firefighter asked.

"The same way we came in," Joaquin answered.

"You mean we have to climb over those . . . again?"

Beth turned toward the opening. "Yep. *Aquí,* Pan. Let's go."

The firefighter's face was edged with green. He sat on the pavement, his head between his knees.

"You okay?" Beth asked, and he nodded.

It was a common reaction, but it never failed to surprise her. This man was a paramedic; gruesome realities were his daily bread. Yet somehow the sight of so many bodies always took its toll on those new to disaster. Even some of the firefighters had no conception of what the weight and force of crashing concrete loosed by an earthquake can do to the human body. Many are reduced to wet spots with bone slivers—not recognizable as human beings at all. Other bodies are twisted, or pummeled to a pulp, or torn into parts. It was a sight to which Beth had numbed herself.

"How many body locations did you and Pan mark?" Joaquin asked.

"Seventeen."

"Good. There were only twenty people missing."

What a terrible measure of success, Beth thought.

"Domino's stood us up again," Carol said as they queued to board the bus for camp that night.

"Yep. We get freeze-dried food eaten dry. Yum."

Carol laughed. "I'd give up a five-course dinner for one bath, slathers of toothpaste, and water to rinse. . . ."

"Stop!" Beth itched at the reminder. How many days now without a bath? Two traveling, four in Armenia. *Six days?* At least this morning she'd managed to change her clothes, but her pants stood up on their own.

Rat-tat-tat-tatta-tatta. The noise bounced from the ruins around them. Beth grabbed Carol's arm. "That was a machine gun!"

A Soviet guard grinned at the women. He held up his own automatic, and pretended to fire. "Rats. Shoot rats."

"The four- or two-legged kind?" Beth whispered as she and Carol jumped into the bus. No one answered.

TWO ALIVE

Day Five: December 15, 5:30 A.M.

An oversized outline of Lenin's profile adorned the ruined billboard next to the partially excavated apartments. A few of the walls were still intact. Wooden stairs inside indicated some were multilevel. One could even see into kitchens.

Beth liked "Lenin's Head" apartments—as she promptly dubbed it—because it was promising for survivors.

"Come on," Ralph called. "This is a good place to get in."

He climbed through a window and swung down on steel lengths of rebars until he dropped ten feet to the floor below. Panda eyed him for a moment, then launched herself into his waiting arms.

"Oof," Ralph puffed, falling backward with ninety-five pounds of white German shepherd sprawled on his chest.

Beth dangled, then eased down. Pan trotted immediately to the wooden stairs, and poked her head underneath. Her mistress dropped to her knees and trailed behind.

"See anything?" Ralph asked

"Not yet, but I hear water running."

Beth flicked on her head lamp, and wormed farther. "Lots of gaps," she reported.

The dog belly-crawled to the edge of a chasm thirty feet deep. She nudged Beth and her entire head disappeared into the breach. The shepherd wanted to go down.

"No. *Aquí.*" Beth backpedaled to Ralph. "I think she's got a live one."

"Where's Joulie? I'll tell her to get the workmen here. You continue on task."

Not long after, Panda snuffled along the top floor of Lenin's Head. Suddenly, she rammed her nose into the tilted partition in front of her. Her claws scrabbled at the wall, and she barked.

"What does that mean?" asked Ralph.

"I don't know," Beth answered. "She never barks. Get Ed and Grief here to confirm. She may have another live one."

Within minutes, Grief and his giant of a master had reached Panda's alert. The black-and-tan furrowed wildly.

"Time to call the heavy-rescue guys," Ed crowed.

"That's what I thought."

"I'll stay here, and start digging out."

"Okay, Ed. There's an opening to the floor below up ahead. Let's see if Panda turns up another surprise."

"Whoa," Beth cried as she slipped on loose gravel covering a tilted floor. "We have to go easy here, Pan."

The shepherd ignored her, and tried to squeeze into the ravaged kitchen beyond.

"*¡Basta!* Stop!" Beth ordered, and grabbed Pan's haunches, yanking the dog backward. "Let me check it out first."

Beth slithered forward and sized up the layout. "Looks stable enough. *Ven, perra.*" Panda shot forward and disappeared. They were directly under Ed and Grief by now.

Pan's china-dish eyes and pink nose announced her reappearance. Her whole body was quivering. "Another live one? Same one as upstairs, I'll bet. Let's tell the others."

Beth pushed with her elbows, propelling herself backward out of the aperture. She stood at last. Panda was already swimming up the pile to the top floor.

Without warning, the rubble broke loose from under her paws. Fist-sized clumps of concrete, hard-hitting chunks of wood, shards of glass, and rods of steel avalanched on top of Beth. She was trapped—to her knees. "My Lord."

Panda wheeled at the sound of her voice, and plunged toward her mistress, inadvertently triggering a new surge of wreckage. "*¡Basta!*" Beth yelled.

Panda froze, suspended above her. The scree stabilized, but now Beth was buried to the waist. "*Vamos,* Pan," Beth commanded. "Go."

The shepherd spun, picked her way to the top and disappeared. Beth didn't move; she barely dared to breathe. She could be buried alive.

A confused babble of voices preceded the rescue party. Brown, craggy faces peered over the broken lip of the floor above. Panda shouldered her way between two Armenians, and watched her mistress intently. One man swung his leg onto the debris. Pebbles snowballed toward the trapped woman.

Beth lifted two hands, palms toward them. "Stop." She wasn't the only one in danger. If someone were breathing in the pit behind her, this cascade could kill them.

Think! She had to think. Panda had been able to get out by dog-paddling. Maybe she could do the same.

Beth laid her body on the shifting mass, displacing her weight. Rocks clipped her face, and she stilled. Her leg was bent in the press of the debris, but it wasn't packed tight enough to be trapped.

With infinitesimal exertion, she rotated her left hip. It moved. Yes! Inch by painful inch—her thigh came free; her knee; at last her foot.

Now the right leg. Her bruised hip was on fire, but she kept moving, biting her lip to concentrate, until she was able to pull clear.

She dared a glance up. The Armenians were perfectly quiet, perfectly still, coiled for action. "No," she whispered.

. Slowly, Beth rolled up the pile. With every slip of stone, she stopped, let her heart calm. The knife-sharp buildup breached the protection of her heavy clothes, biting into her skin like a rack of nails.

Her head pounded. Still she rolled, waited, rolled again. Only a few feet more. She pushed on. A dozen hands reached toward her, closing on her coveralls, her belt, her coat, and lifted her to safety.

Panda sniffed her face and down her arms. "I'm all right, Pan. Really, I am."

"Are you sure?" Joulie demanded. "I was scared to death."

Beth nodded. "Me, too."

"There's a crane on the way. They'll find whoever's down there."

Beth could only nod again. The taste of being trapped made her feel more empathy than ever toward the victims of this disaster. "I hope they do."

Ed Johnson weaved through the various international teams on Lenin's Head until he located Beth. "Bad news. You know those live alerts Panda and Grief scented? They were live, all right. It was the French rescue guys, working the far side of the building."

Beth's newfound optimism drained. "Thanks, Ed."

The tall American patted his dog. "I know how you feel."

Sporadic gunfire cracked throughout the city. The sound followed the team in their searches, startling them, breaking their concentration. It chased them as they bused to their camp that night.

"There's talk of riots, looting, and civil disturbances, but I don't know," Ralph said. "Every time I've asked one of our State Department people, they just shrug and get these worried expressions."

"Look," Beth exclaimed, pointing out the window toward an intersection. A company of soldiers toting bazookas, flanked by three tanks and a dozen Soviet army jeeps, marched quick-time in front of them. "What's going on? The troops are multiplying faster than the coffins."

The camp crawled with Armenians that night, many begging for medical help. Equipment was primitive. One doctor set the leg of a man while he lay on the trunk of a car. Others stitched open wounds. The Americans dispensed antibiotics and painkillers.

But all had not come begging aid.

A woman held out some bread and a small bottle of cognac to Beth.

"No, no." Beth stepped back, trying to resist without insulting the generosity of the gift giver.

The Armenian pushed her tokens into Beth's hands. "Thank you." She bent to Panda, patted her on the head, and gave her a candy. "Thank you."

"Our dogs are going to get fat on all these sweets." Brooke laughed as Buster gulped down her offering. "And have you ever tasted anything like this bread? Better'n pizza any day."

Ralph stood on an empty crate in the middle of the crowd, and clapped for attention. "Listen up. Listen up, people. Word from HQ is we leave tomorrow." A babble of questions bombarded him, and he threw up his hands. "Does it have anything to do with the troop buildup? I haven't a clue. They don't tell me anything. All I know is it's time to move."

The news didn't comfort anybody. There was still so much to do. "Look on the bright side. Maybe we can finally get a bath," Brooke said as she and Beth headed toward their tents.

A bath. That sounded too wonderful to be true. It had been eight days since Beth's skin had touched soap or water, and the crud that accumulated all over her could be peeled off in sheets.

Joaquin strolled by. "Hey. Remember the dogs' alert at Lenin's Head?" he asked Beth.

"Yeah. Don't remind me. The French team."

"Maybe not. After we left, they found two boys."

Beth grabbed his arm. "You kidding me?"

"Nope. We aren't getting credit for the find, but who cares? Pretty good news, huh?"

Two alive. She held out her bottle of cognac. "How about a toast? To the people of Armenia."

"I'll raise a glass to that."

HOME AGAIN

The entire U.S. rescue team was gathered again, this time in the White House. President Ronald Reagan walked to a central podium, smiling and chatting with the strike force as he worked the room. When the crowd quieted, he spoke.

"Thanks to people like you here today, the Armenians have not had to face the tragedy alone. You conveyed what was a truly universal message, one for us all to remember at this time of year, that every life is infinitely precious, a gift from God."

"The Armenians are the true heroes," Beth whispered to Ralph as the president continued.

"You're right about that."

The State Department

The chandeliers sparkled in the muted elegance of the Georgian room. Buffet tables were scattered here and there, vivid with flowers but oddly empty of food.

Joaquin bellied up to a table. "This 'hero' stuff ain't all bad, is it, Beth? But I wonder what's for lunch?"

Just at that moment, the double doors burst open and a parade of people, each holding steaming Domino's boxes, marched down the center of the room.

"Did anyone order pizza?" an aide asked.

The rescue workers who had shared the camp in Armenia—and the nightly joke—burst out laughing. "Yes!" they yelled.

"What'd I tell you?" Joaquin exclaimed. "Let's eat."

Beth Barkley decided then and there that the State Department knew how to throw a party.

PART THREE

SEASONED VETERAN

CHAPTER 12

TRANSITIONS

Mud slides, wildfires, floods, hurricanes, earthquakes. Natural disasters. They happen; they are non-negotiable, and there's nothing anyone can do about nature's rage.

In 1988, the ponderous bulk of the U.S. government finally moved, struck by the light. Disaster can't be prevented; the fallout can only be alleviated. And planning for this fallout must be effected on a national level. As a result of this thinking, the Federal Emergency Management Agency (FEMA) was tasked to respond. One of its first orders of business was to incorporate search and rescue into its disaster planning—including the use of search dogs.

Beth was called upon to write some of the urban search-and-rescue guidelines for the fledgling directive, and was recruited as a member of the newly formed task force from Virginia. It meant many more hours of classes, seminars, instructing, and field work so that the new FEMA teams could operate as smooth-functioning units—groups that could immediately respond to a federal emergency, either at home or for OFDA abroad.

FEMA used the Incident Command System, similar to the chain of command practiced by firefighters of the National Park Service, which had become second nature

to Beth. She and her dogs could now slip into the struc-
ture of any other team anywhere in the United States. She
became aware of how easily the inside jargon of police
and military slipped off her tongue, and realized with a
shock how far Beth Barkley had come since that first
search for the Boy Scouts at Quantico, six years before.

But she pushed ever further. The seasoned professional was invited, and made it a point to attend, the
Trench Rescue Operations Team refresher classes held
once a month by the Fairfax County Fire Department.
Before long, she added chainsaw and jackhammer operation to her growing reservoir of knowledge.

Through it all, Sirius shone. Beth allowed Panda to
participate, because she still enjoyed the activity, but it
was on Siri that Beth now relied. She took the new dog
all over the country, and he learned like lightning. But
one habit of his nagged at Beth. Siri would begin a search
with great enthusiasm, but would weary, stop, and lie
down. Moments later, he'd be back on task.

It worried her, but she couldn't see anything wrong.
Siri was beautifully fit at 105 pounds; he never showed
pain, and was always eager to work.

Not too long after the shepherd began his mysterious
behavior, Joanne Chanyi and Sharon Mann, the Canadian
women who had been responsible for breeding him,
came to visit Beth. After a dinner of roast chicken with
the works, the women relaxed with glasses of Armenian
cognac. Panda and Siri sprawled at their feet like twin
deities.

"I told you he was a love of a pup," Sharon said, nod-
ding toward Sirius.

"Oh, he is. We're having a ball."

"How's he doing with his search work?" Joanne asked.

"He's been doing fine, up till now. But there's a bit of a problem, and it's worrying me." Beth described Siri's behavior, and both women looked perplexed.

"I made a video for FEMA of one of his training routines. Would you like to see it?"

"Yeah. Maybe we can spot something," Joanne encouraged.

The women relaxed and watched Siri move like a dancer over an obstacle course.

Suddenly, Joanne sat up rod straight and stared. "Play that back."

Obligingly, Beth ran the portion of the tape again.

"Don't you see it?"

"What?" Beth asked.

"I can't see anything," Sharon exclaimed.

"He's limping. Back left leg."

Beth played the tape again. This time, both she and Sharon spotted the slight favoring Siri gave to his left side.

"I think that's your problem," Joanne stated. "He's hurt."

Dr. Cockrill waved Beth into his office. Siri's X rays were illuminated by the bright square of light. "See? He's got a cracked femur. And another fracture lower down. It's hairline, but it's hurting him. I'm surprised he never let you know."

"No. Not once. What can be done?"

"First thing, Beth, you'll have to retire him. He can't work in this condition."

She thought of the eager puppy she'd grown to love. "Whatever I have to do, Doc. You know that."

"There's one more thing. He's too heavy. You'll have to get him down to about ninety pounds. Then his leg won't bother him so much."

"I can do that," Beth promised.

That very day, she invented the "green bean" diet. Half of Siri's food was canned green beans—the dog loved it. Soon, he weighed in at a mere eighty-nine pounds, and his limp disappeared.

Beth listened to the doctor's words, and Siri worked no more. She didn't believe there would ever be other dogs like Panda and Sirius, but she called Sharon Mann.

"I think it's time Siri had a brother or sister, don't you?" Sharon asked. "I have Seka. I'll call Joanne. Pancho is still a great sire."

"The same sire and bitch as Sirius. I couldn't ask for anything better."

In April of 1990, Beth got the call. Sharon had a pup.

CHAPTER 13

MEANT TO BE

April 1990

Had she forgotten anything? For the third time Beth ran a quick last-minute check. Extra sweater for the colder Winnipeg nights; cashier's check in Canadian currency; toiletries; change of clothes. All she had to do in the morning was get up, grab her pack and puppy kennel, and head to the airport.

The insistent buzz of the doorbell sounded through the house. Beth smiled; 7:55 P.M. Gayle was late again, but what did it matter? Bless her heart. Gayle Arrington was special.

Like Beth, Gayle loved dogs—especially white German shepherds. Indeed, Gayle was the editor of the White German Shepherd Club newsletter. The two women had met for an interview after Beth's return from Armenia. They had become so close they referred to themselves as "dog-in-laws."

Beth threw open the door to see Gayle's pleasant face. A woman of generous proportions, whose thin, gray hair hung in soft waves past her shoulder, pushed into the house. Her "in-law" looked tired tonight. She'd been putting in too much overtime at Customs lately, and it was showing.

"I've got your favorite lamb stew for dinner and a nice bottle of Chardonnay," Beth chatted as she led the way into the living room.

Panda and Siri immediately pounced on the familiar figure, barking in welcome. "Down now, down." Gayle tried to sound severe. She pulled open her voluminous carpetbag and extracted two thick dog bones. The shepherds strained forward. Gayle placed one in each eager mouth and the dogs scurried into their respective night kennels to gobble them in peace.

"You do love to spoil them, don't you?" Beth teased, bringing them two glasses of chilled wine. "To the new pup, Sirius Too," she toasted.

"Isn't that just like Sharon to name her after Siri?"

The singsong chime of the telephone interrupted them. "Who could that be?" Beth wondered, frowning. "Go make yourself comfortable." She nodded toward Gayle's favorite armchair and picked up the receiver.

It was Sharon Mann. "I've got bad news." Her Canadian brogue was clipped, too fast. "I took your pup to the vet for her health certificate and he detected a heart murmur." The breeder hesitated and her next words came out slow, sad, apologetic. "He says she'll be lucky to see a first birthday. I'm sorry, Beth."

"What's the matter?" Gayle mouthed.

Beth covered the mouthpiece of the telephone with her free hand. "The pup's very sick."

Gayle's broad face creased into concern. "Oh, Beth."

"I'm glad I caught you before you left," Sharon said.

"Yeah, it won't do any good to come up now."

"Wait a minute," Gayle interjected. "Your ticket's nonrefundable. Go anyway."

Beth hesitated. Gayle put down her wine, rose, and

grabbed the handset. "Hi, Sharon? Gayle. How you doing? Not so good, eh?" She listened. "You were? Well then, she'll be there tomorrow as planned." She hung up the telephone and leveled her gaze at Beth.

"You're going," Gayle said. "Sharon was looking forward to seeing you. Besides, it's only for the weekend. You could do with the break."

"You don't look so good yourself, Gayle."

"Just tired, Beth. Just tired." The familiar grin made her beautiful. "Besides, Panda and Siri will give me plenty of rest."

"Sure they will," Beth said.

The next morning saw her in coach class to Canada.

Sharon's ranch-style home was exactly as she'd imagined: large, attractive rooms filled with deep-cushioned sofas, most occupied with a contentedly snoring canine. There were the occasional toys on the floor, but the house did not appear to be the home of six white shepherds that is was.

The breeder led the way to the immaculate kitchen, where a pup was curled up in the middle of a red-plaid doggy cushion. Her fluffy white body looked small and vulnerable in the middle of all that color. Amber eyes met Beth's as the visitor squatted beside her. The pup struggled to feet unsteady with sleep and nudged a cold nose into her outstretched fingers.

"Pick her up," Sharon instructed, averting her eyes as the pup anointed the new face with wet swipes of her tongue. Now Beth could hear the painfully loud thump of an irregular heartbeat. "She's a sweet thing, but no good for what you want."

Sharon was a decent human being, but breeding dogs was her business. The pup wouldn't be ill treated, but then it wouldn't get much attention while it lived. The golden eyes that reminded Beth so much of her own Sirius melted into pure puppy love.

Beth heard her own words and wondered where they came from. "I'd like to take her. I've got lots of room; she wouldn't be in the way, and perhaps your next litter . . ." She did have extra space, but she should know better. The vet bills for a healthy dog were bad enough; this little love could have her eating peanut butter and jelly forever. Yet she held the puppy close. She didn't know why, but Beth felt Sirius Too had to go home with her.

"You don't have to take her for that. I'll call you again when I think I have the right dog."

Sharon was giving her an out. Beth carefully lowered the pup into her bed and stood up.

"That's not the reason." How did she explain that it just felt like the right thing to do?

Sharon looked Beth up and down as though assessing her for breeding stock. "Follow me," she finally ordered.

The woman strode ahead down a short hallway and opened the door at the end. The room was lined with bookcases, filled with old titles long forgotten. The late afternoon sun dappled across pinewood floors in slanting golden rays. Not a stick of furniture decorated the space; the room was empty, save for a five-foot-square wire dog pen that dominated the center. Three barking canines within immediately rushed to the limit of their enclosure.

Two of them were normal white German shepherd puppies, around ten pounds, noisy, and curious. The third looked as though it had taken up most of its mother's womb. Comparisons with linebackers immediately came to mind. The dog even acted like a football player, lumbering up behind his siblings and shouldering them aside like so many bubbles.

"Guess which one's the boy?" Sharon asked.

"That would be too easy."

"He's called Czar. 'Czar the Terrible,' actually. He's promised to the Toronto Police Department."

"Seems like a good place for him."

The women watched the roly-poly tumbling of the pups in companionable silence. "I think you should take him."

"But . . ."

"Hear me out. Czar's a handful, yes. Rambunctious, hard to control. But with the right person he'd make a great search dog. You're a pro, Beth. Take him; he'll be a good dog for you."

"But the Toronto Police?"

Sharon grinned. "They'll wait for my next litter."

Gayle was waiting for her with two freshly groomed adult dogs and a takeout pizza. "You brought the sick one!" she exclaimed as Beth dragged two kennels into the house. "Oh, you poor little thing," she murmured, nuzzling Too against her cheek.

"I couldn't leave her. Sharon said she won't last the year."

"Well, that makes two of us."

Beth was still thinking about the pup. "What?"

"I said, that makes two of us."

"That's not funny, Gayle."

Gayle put the white fluff ball on her lap and looked straight at her "in-law."

"I didn't tell you, but I had some tests taken. The doc called me Friday. I've got uterine cancer, Beth. Bad. I have about a year at most." She continued to scratch the pup behind the ears. For her part, Sirius Too pushed with all her puny might against the gentle pressure of Gayle's fingers. "Let me keep this one, Beth. You're gonna have your hands full with that monster you've brought home. Too and I can comfort each other."

"The vet bills will kill you."

Gayle smiled. "It seems I'm dying already. Remember?"

"I'm so sorry, I didn't mean . . ."

"I know you didn't, but *I* mean it. Let me have this pup."

"You can have anything I've got."

"Be careful what you offer," Gayle teased.

Beth took care of Too until after her in-law's surgery. After Gayle and Too officially became a couple, Beth called every day until Gayle finally told her to stop acting like a mother hen. "Too's so funny," she'd say, neatly changing the subject, then spend the next half hour relating how Too had kept her up half the night playing before going to sleep on her belly. Beth didn't blame the pup. She'd often thought Gayle's belly would make a wonderful pillow.

Her friend never mentioned the weekly vet visits; the fear when Too's heart almost gave out; the expensive medication. And it took Beth a while to realize how skillfully Gayle steered their conversation away from her cancer.

The next few months ran away for Beth, Panda, Siri, and Czar. For Gayle and Too, also, so it seemed. Gayle gave up her job at Customs, and she and the pup took to visiting children's hospitals and senior citizens. Too was so popular, folks would buy her doggy treats and send letters to her. Their visits, Gayle often said, were the difference between living and "living death" for the people they touched.

Beth watched the year-mark approach and pass; then eighteen months. How did a dying twosome manage to look so good?

Then came the call.

"Beth," her friend said solemnly, and she knew it was bad.

"Gayle . . ."

A yell blasted the line between them. "Beth, I'm in remission! Not a damn cancer cell anywhere! And I'm supposed to be dead, girl!" Beth felt a rush of such love, such relief. "And Too told me she ain't going anywhere, either. I mean it's how long now?"

"One year, ten months," Beth mumbled. Three days and eight hours, she could have added.

She thought long and hard that day. What had compelled her to bring the little sick pup home against all reason? It didn't matter. All Beth knew as her head hit the pillow that night was that she was meant to go to Canada, meant to bring back a sick pup to a sick friend. It was one of the best rescues she'd ever made in her life.

She also wondered if the "monster" pup, Czar, was preordained. She would find out soon enough.

CHAPTER 14

THE PUPPY
FROM HELL

If Beth had not known better, she would have concluded that Czar had been sent to torment her for some grievous sin from a past life. "Sit!" she commanded. "Sit still, you silly thing. How do you expect me to doctor you?"

Czar plopped on his haunches, his big tongue panting happily as he gazed at his mistress, totally oblivious to the stream of blood sliding over his muzzle to puddle on the grass in front of him. Panda stood to one side, oozing impatient disbelief, a decided look of "nothing good ever came out of Nazareth" stamped on her face as she watched the young bumpkin.

Beth sighed, rinsed her cotton clear of the red liquid, and held it over the wound on Czar's nose. It wasn't a very deep gash; in a few seconds she'd be able to dab some antibiotic cream on it, and it would heal naturally.

Only her Czar could attack his training with such enthusiastic abandon. What other dog would take off like a rocket, look over his shoulder for his person's approval, and galumph smack into one of only five trees bordering their training area?

Not even Panda and Siri's calm could influence this hyperactive bundle of energy. Beth would try. As befitted her oldest dog's seniority, she would send Pan on ahead with Czar trailing a few seconds later. That way, the youngster could learn something—she hoped. It never worked.

Czar had no respect. Instead of keeping a discreet distance as Beth commanded, he would rush Panda's rear and nudge her haunches, all the time nipping at her heels and yammering his incessant "Yaa. Yaa. Yaa."

Panda, as Royal Victoria before her, was not amused. She became ever more regal, finally reverting to her old Empress of the Pack habits. She would sweep around and crunch Czar firmly on his black snout. "Yip!" Czar would cry, and return to Beth, tail between his legs. It didn't take long before Czar bowed to Panda with the deference the elderly dog already commanded from Siri.

But now it had been two years since Beth had brought Czar home; something had to be done with the crazy animal. There was one person in search and rescue for whom Beth had the highest respect. Andy Rebmann was a retired Connecticut State Trooper who'd been training dogs for more than two decades. Andy had developed the definitive method of teaching dogs to distinguish minute amounts of dead matter that could be used for evidence. He'd formulated a substance, with Sigma Chemical Company, called "Cadaverine." Cadaver search was advanced training.

By taking Czar to Rebmann's course, Beth would be instructing the shepherd "ass-backward," as Andy would say. But by now Beth was ready to try anything with the "gargantua" of a dog named Czar.

CHAPTER 15

BONDING CZAR

August 1993

Andy Rebmann's course was being held in Bozrah, a small rural community near Norwich, Connecticut. Its claim to fame is that the farmers thereabouts raise the best chickens in North America. They also spread the chicken manure on the surrounding fields, which gives rise to another kind of notoriety; Bozrah has the biggest, fattest flies on the East Coast. Some wags swear the Bozrah fly is the state bird of Connecticut.

Czar didn't know what to make of the strange odors that drifted through the open windows. His scent receptors worked overtime, and he looked at Beth as if this were wondrous indeed.

The dog got another shock when they checked into the Norwich Hotel on the outskirts of town. Czar had never been to a hotel before. He padded in cocky enough, then pulled up short as if he'd run into an electric fence.

His nose hit the floor with a loud sniffle. Czar followed the scent to the bathroom. A minute later, he was on the bed with his muzzle stuck in the coverlet. He bounded from bed to floor, chair to window, then ran at Beth, his eyes huge. She could read his amazement. *Do you know how many people have been in here?*

Beth was in a good mood, looking forward to being a student for a change. Andy ran a very intense two weeks with only six people. Beth knew well you never stop learning in search work. She, as well as Czar, would glean a lot from this course.

They were to meet in the upstairs social hall of the Bozrah Volunteer Fire Department. But there was no instructor to greet the group the next morning. Instead, a terse note tacked to the door gave them their first assignment. "Find 'Matilda,' " it read. Four hand-drawn maps of the surrounding swampy woods were stapled to the bottom. Nobody had a clue who "Matilda" might be, but everyone figured that Andy wanted to see how they performed in the field before he started work with them.

Beth paired with another veteran. Donna Johnson was from Boston. Her shepherd Zenturo and Panda were old pals. Zenturo sniffed the two-year-old, then nuzzled Czar with affection. "Do you think he can smell Pan?" Donna asked.

The women worked their dogs on opposite sides of the farm road. All was going as it should when Beth heard a racket that would wake a hedgehog in hibernation. She tucked into a run and splashed through the knee-high purple asters that crowded the floor of the old-growth forest. In a small glen dappled with sunlight, Czar had found the plastic body that was Matilda.

The ivory mannequin dangled from the solid branch of a paper-white birch about five feet above him. Czar couldn't compute the entity that looked and smelled like a human, and moved, yet had no life. His head tilted so far back Beth thought he might topple over.

She chuckled. That was enough insult for Czar. He lunged and smacked heavily against the belly of the model. Matilda swayed like one of Circe's sirens. The shepherd growled, backed off, and charged again. Now it was Matilda's turn to soar. She jerked skyward and caught on a limb ten feet above.

"Oh, no, Czar." Beth groaned.

Andy strolled into the clearing. "That's the first time that's happened." He roughed the fur on the shepherd's haunches. "Good confirmation. Healthy coat. How you doing, Beth?" He smiled at the woman he'd met at conferences over the years.

Andy never changed. His ancient Connecticut trooper's cap was still pushed back on a head of rumpled dun hair. If anything, the deep valleys that bisected his hangdog face made him resemble his beloved bloodhounds more than ever. "Sorry, Andy. I think I've got Dr. Czar and Mr. Hyde here."

"Nah. I put 'Cadaverine' scent in Matilda's chest cavity. Your dog recognized the smell of something dead, he just didn't understand what it was. He was protecting you. I'm glad I didn't have Matilda in the classroom. He'd have eaten her."

Donna and Zenturo joined them. The three people stared up at the model.

"What we have to decide now," Andy deadpanned, "is who's gonna make the climb up and get the damn thing down?" He peered at Beth, and the look said it all.

After the first unfortunate encounter with Matilda, Czar seemed to settle down. He was still the only dog to crawl onto his mistress's lap during class time. It was a precarious perch, and Beth always pushed him off and gave a stern "sit" order. The shepherd tipped his head, his face bright with surprise, a perfect imitation of "Who, me?" that reduced the whole class to laughter.

Czar still yattered like a goofy fool when he socialized with the other dogs, and didn't think it unseemly to sniff the one female's nether region. But when Beth ordered *"napu,"* the Seminole Indian word for death she'd decided to use, Czar seemed to understand the seriousness of the training. He set his mind to the mission with the finesse of a warrior. Even daylong tramps through Bozrah's famous chicken-fertilized fields didn't deter Czar's determined nose from sniffing fully on the inert air for the "napu" he was supposed to seek out.

As the first week passed, Czar learned so well that while Beth studied she allowed him to snooze the afternoons away with his head in her lap. But she drew the line when they went to bed. "Absolutely not," she told the dog when he belly-slithered under the coverlet to get next to her. At home, that was where Panda liked to sleep.

It was on a sweltering Tuesday forenoon that Czar stole his mistress's heart. Andy had planned their first water search at a farm pond. First thing that morning the trooper had wrapped the "Cadaverine" capsule in gauze, put it in a net bag, weighted it with a rock, and thrown it into the lake.

In the afternoon Andy decreed that it was Czar's turn in the spotlight. Everybody watched as Beth walked the shepherd around the body of water. Her instructions were to lag behind, and let her dog work alone.

Czar loped off on command, but he kept running back to circle Beth as if to chide her for being slow. *"Napu. Napu,"* she ordered. "Go, Czar," she added for good measure. And the dog reluctantly cantered ahead.

To throw his "scent" into the water, Andy had stood on a lichen-covered boulder directly across from the observation point. Beth watched her dog reach the launch spot and scramble up. If Czar detected the sunken "cadaverine," it would be a major coup.

But the shepherd was nonplussed—or just enjoying the view. An airy monarch butterfly chose that moment to flutter in front of the dog's nose. *Shoot*, Beth thought. But Czar stilled in dreamy concentration as the monarch teased his periphery.

It was something beautiful to see, the dog's fascination for the insect working the hushed air above him. He was truly majestic. *Where is my camera?*

The butterfly grew tired of the game. Czar watched it disappear into the summer greenness of a neighboring oak. At the same time a 747 drew its way across the cloudless sky. Czar traced its hazy contrail until it, too, evaporated.

The dog shook himself back to reality, and stared into the water below him. With gold-medal precision, Czar dove. He spoiled it somewhat when he splashed into the lake with a loud belly-flop, but Beth was exultant. "Find it, Czar. You can do it." Even Andy couldn't guess the "Cadaverine" location, but Czar worked it like a pro. He paddled forward, and a bark and eager snapping at the surface told the tale. Czar had found it.

A cheer erupted from his human companions. Andy beamed like a proud father. Czar would be lavishly praised indeed for this "find."

A happy if exhausted Beth tumbled into bed that night. Czar sat on the floor and gazed longingly at the place beside her as he had every night since their arrival.

Beth scooted to one side of the mattress. She smiled

and patted the covers. With a joyous bark, Czar clambered on board and snuggled against her. Before a half hour passed he was snoring happily into her ear. Beth turned over and felt Czar wriggle his body against her back—he wasn't going to let her get away. She closed her eyes and let sleep take over.

CHAPTER 16

ADIOS, MI AMIGA

October 1993

Panda was growing old now. She'd suffered for her work, and Beth didn't want pain to be her only payback for heroism. So she made sure her best friend warmed her old bones in sun-washed bliss, basking in golden squares of light that heated the floor near a wood-burning stove.

Occasionally, if the day was fine, Panda would venture forth with her mistress and relive the glory days. At the call of a thrush on a woodland trail she would swivel her eyes to catch Beth's. *Remember other days like this?*

"Si, amiga mia," Beth would answer softly.

As Panda's time grew shorter, it became less idyllic. When her pitted lungs struggled for every rasping breath, Beth would cradle her head and shoulders on pillows in her lap. On the solitary night watch her mistress would whisper stories of their great adventures, watching Pan's ears twitch to catch every nuance of the beloved voice. She would knead tired muscles to coax Panda to close her eyes. Never did Beth begrudge one lost hour of sleep. She'd gladly give it all for time with Panda.

Yet love and care could not hold back the inevitable.

With the dying of the year, the dog lost ground. One day when Beth and Czar returned from a search in West Virginia, Panda didn't greet them. It was a ritual the dog had never failed to perform since that fateful wedding party so many years before. The old dog lay near the stove, and could barely lift her head when her mistress knelt beside her. "No, Pan. *Por favor.* I'm not ready to say good-bye."

Panda's tail brushed the floor, and her beautiful face seemed sympathetic to her mistress's distress; yet it was resolved. The woman stayed beside her for untold minutes, coming to grips with the truth. Beth could not, would not, allow her friend to suffer.

She called Jean Hooks, the vet, to alert her, and eased the limp, white form into her car. Czar and Siri rode along, "the Terrible" subdued for once in his rambunctious life. Every now and then one of them would venture a soothing lick to Panda's paw—the only spot they could manage to reach.

Jean and her assistant met them at the car. There was no need to hurt Panda by moving her any more. Mere minutes it took, and she suffered no longer.

"Adios, mi amiga," Beth choked. *"Perrita de mi corazón."*

That night was chilled, misty with rain. Beth wrapped her girl in blankets, unable to bear the idea of her being cold, then buried Panda with her beloved shabrack under the shepherd's favorite oak.

The next morning, a somber Czar and Siri led their mistress to Panda's grave, which they had already partially dug up. "I can't bring her back," she tried to explain to the young dogs. Concerned that they would again try to unearth their mentor's body, Beth bought mums and winter pansies. Pan had loved flowers. She troweled and planted until her fingernails were torn and black with dirt and her knees raw. Still, Beth couldn't stop. Panda had liked to watch finches and sparrows in the spring, so Beth set a birdbath under the tree. She added whimsical stone statues and a bench for quiet reflection.

It became a lovingly tended spot to honor a valiant, beloved spirit.

Panda's garden.

CHAPTER 17

HEALING

Like a first love, Panda would never be forgotten. But, as another cliché comforts, time passes, especially if one fills it. Beth became ever more involved in her chosen volunteer work. She founded her own nonprofit training group, Search Services America, and immediately attracted some of the police and firefighters she'd worked with in the past.

Siri was now a loving friend, certified in pet therapy, who greeted his mistress as if she were Ulysses returned from a quest when she came home. Czar was as obstreperous as ever, but Beth let him have his head for the most part. She well knew that the drive and intensity that may not make a dog a good pet was essential for a great search dog.

Just a little while before, Beth had returned from teaching a seven-day course for FEMA at Camp Atterbury, Indiana. Beth would instruct, while next door twenty-nine of the thirty dogs in the program would quietly await their persons' return. But not *her* dog. Czar barked and yowled and nattered until finally Beth had had enough. She marched into the adjoining room and stuck her face in his. "Shut up," she ordered.

But Czar proved his worth on the second evening.

Beth took him for a walk to unwind. Suddenly, the dog's tail was wagging faster than a hummingbird's wings. He barked and stared into the bushes at the edge of the woods. Beth was tired. "What is it this time, Czar?"

Ninety-six pounds of dog jumped and planted his paws on his mistress's chest. "Woof! Woof!" Czar barked so loudly in her face, he sprayed her with spit.

Maybe something *was* wrong. "Find 'em," Beth ordered, and Czar shot off.

"Damn and shit!" came the loud expletive. A young man, crossbow slung across his back, slunk out of the bushes with his hands in the air. Czar had taken a prisoner.

"He won't hurt you," Beth said, trying to keep a straight face. "He thought you might be lost. Good boy, Czar. Good dog."

"I was trying to *hide*. The Navy SEALs are conducting maneuvers out here." The boy lowered his hands. "He sure is big, ma'am."

Then he realized his behavior. He looked at Beth, at the VDES and FEMA insignias on her wool jacket, and must have thought she was somebody he should salute. He straightened, stared ahead, and snapped his hand to his forehead.

"Ease up, friend." Beth laughed. "I'm not the admiral."

The boy dropped his arm. "No, ma'am."

"So, the navy's here, too? I'm teaching a training class with dogs."

"That might be dangerous, ma'am. Some of us are carrying live weapons."

Beth took notes on the SEALs' coordinates and vowed to keep her own band well away. Thanks to Czar, they were spared a possible "incident."

Yes, Czar was on his way to being one of the best. Like Panda before him he would ride the wind, his dark nose air-scenting across the miles in search after search. Under Beth's tutelage the shepherd also became proficient in trailing, a crucial skill in evidence work.

But not since Andy Rebmann's class had Czar experienced any further practice in cadaver work. Maybe that was why, the night before Independence Day, Beth said "yes" when requested to do a cadaver search instead of enjoying barbecue and fireworks. That, and the fact that Ross, the detective who asked for her help, was a member of her newly formed Search Services America.

CHAPTER 18

DRUG KING OF
THE NORTHEAST

July 4th

It was a drug deal gone sour. The two kingpins were known to the Prince William County police. These boys were not street-level hustlers; they were the big-money operators. "The beef between them must have been pretty heavy duty," Ross surmised.

As far as the Narcotics Division could construct the crime, the two had met in typical Mafia-movie fashion on a lonely road, and hadn't been able to iron out their differences. One was never seen again. A year later the Drug Enforcement Agency had the survivor locked up in Lorton prison on other charges. The suspect had boasted, "I offed the mother—— with a hammer. The suckers can look. They ain't goin' to find that skull."

Ross laid it out to Beth. "We've narrowed the search to a section of road with a stream running alongside. We found human vertebrae, and we're sure they belong to the slain dealer. But to cinch the case and get a conviction, we need the skull."

"Okay—so?"

"We're stumped. I know it's a holiday tomorrow, but could you and Czar . . . ?"

"Czar loves to work on the Fourth," Beth joked, then got serious. Ross and his yellow lab, Mavrick, were coming along well, and she was proud of their progress. They could turn this into a real training exercise. "Give me the location," she said, all business.

The police had cordoned off three miles of road. Beth was welcomed with smiles when she joined the knot of officers manning the barricade at the south end. "Glad you could make it, Beth," Ross greeted her.

He was waiting with his flop-eared Labrador, his captain, and several other officers connected to the case. Beth was surprised to be introduced to two forensic pathologists from the Smithsonian Institution. "We're in rarefied company today," she murmured to her buddy.

Beth stared down the incline at the slumberous stream with its shallow pools of congealed water. This was where the vertebrae had been found. Classic place to throw a body, per Andy Rebmann's class.

A section of vegetation had been bushwhacked, but on either side of the cleared area the embankments stretched to infinity, overgrown with vines and poison ivy. They could handle that.

What was really on Beth's mind was her hunch that Ross's division hadn't quite come around to taking him seriously when it came to his search work. "Want to be a hero?" she asked.

"What d'you mean?"

"Let Mavrick make the find if it's here. I think the best shot is upstream. Czar and I'll go the other way."

The detective demurred only briefly. Beth could tell he was pleased for the chance. They collected their dogs and took off in opposite directions.

The spring floods had cut deep swaths under the banks

near the road. The heat of Virginia had evaporated all but inches of water in the stream above a bed of mud and sand. Under the heavy summer air the standing pools were still as glass, perfect breeding grounds for the predatory mosquitoes that hung above their surface.

Czar had snuffled his way along the stream's edges for going on an hour. Beth was beginning to question whether they had been called too late. If the marrow had leached out of the bones, neither Mavrick nor Czar would ever find the skull; there would be nothing there for the bacteria to work on. All the scent would be gone.

Slogging along the stream wasn't dangerous, just hot, tedious work. Every quarter of an hour, Beth scooped up a canteen of dirty water and poured it over Czar's head to cool him down. *Only mad dogs and Englishmen go out in the noonday sun—or a nutty woman and her SAR dog.* "I wonder if Ross is having any better luck up his end, Czar?"

Czar had nothing to say.

Up ahead the stream curved. The floods had exposed the roots of a lone weeping willow. They would rest under its shade and Beth would rethink the mission.

But Czar had other ideas. He trotted into the stream where the tree hung over and poked his big head way under the hollowed bank, plunging his face into six inches of water. As Beth drew abreast he lifted his dripping muzzle and nudged her hard in the belly. The dog could barely contain himself. He pranced back and forth, every now and then jabbing under the bank with his nose. Czar had found something very dead.

"Good dog, good dog," she praised effusively and pulled a doggy treat from her pocket. Czar ignored the food and started to paw.

The forensic experts had made it clear they wanted no digging in any suspect areas. Beth quickly grabbed Czar's ruff and pulled him back, again offering the treat. "Stay," she commanded and blocked his way with her body. Czar dropped his backside in the dirty water and watched as Beth tied a big piece of orange flagging tape on a branch.

"*Napu*, Czar. Let's see if there's anything else around here." Czar identified twenty-three other places downstream, although without the excitement of the first. In some places Beth saw bones. Finally the shepherd sat. *That's it*, he said without words. And the dog and his mistress climbed up the embankment to the road.

Ross was not thirty yards away. His face told her he'd had little success. "Retrace my steps," Beth said. "Let's see what Mavrick does."

It took a while for a flushed Ross to come rushing back. "We did it," he yelled. "The forensic experts dug out the skull just where Czar and Mavrick alerted. In the pool under the willow." Beth smiled at the detective's enthusiasm. This was good for Ross and his dog.

Beth and the officers from Narcotics sat fascinated on the stream bank drinking water or Coke while the forensic experts gave them an education.

"Would you like to know how a skull cracks when it's hit by a hammer?" one asked. He had a rapt audience. "This is where the first blow landed. You see how it split the head open?"

Beth grimaced. "Thunk."

"And here is where the second blow hit. But you can see from the damage that it was the first blow that killed him."

Beth enjoyed learning, even about such a gruesome subject. She'd always been curious about all aspects of police evidence work. The holiday was shot anyway. She'd wait around for the photographs.

Beth took Czar to relieve himself while they set up a large cardboard box and perched the skull in the center. The way it sat, stark and bleached, the way the sun bounced off the whiteness of the bones, made it an object of pity. There was nothing frightening in this old nightmare image.

Czar's reaction on the way back from his toilet was a lesson in dog perception. He saw the box from a few yards away and stilled. His ears flattened; he lowered his head, thrust his neck forward, and approached cautiously. Now he could see what he'd scented and Beth could only surmise that to Czar it didn't look right. He could recognize the head as human, even though devoid of life; but what was it doing without a body attached, stuck on the top of a box in the middle of a country road?

Beth remembered the way Czar had gone at Matilda, the "cadaver," and stayed close. But Czar was a more mature dog now. Paw in front of paw he advanced. He sniffed. He walked around the cardboard podium. He sniffed once more, then sat. You couldn't fool him again. This was no plastic mannequin. This was human. Maybe he couldn't quite figure out what it all computed to, but he knew his people smell—alive or dead.

Beth looked up to see Ross and his buddies smile knowingly.

"Good going, boy," said one. "That's the way to do it."

Yes, Czar had done it well. And Beth knew that from

now on a search for the dead would pose no problem for the dog.

Too soon Czar would prove it again.

CHAPTER 19

CLOSURE

Early Spring, 1995

Rain. Hard, solid sheets of cold rain had fallen for a week. It blocked the man's view of turquoise hills bending toward purple-misted valleys. He often watched the sun set over Charlottesville, knowing that Thomas Jefferson had loved the emerald springs softened by blush-white apple blossoms as much as he did.

But today the man wondered if he should build an ark. The thought struck him funny. He turned to share it with his wife of thirty years who was putting a plump chicken in the oven. That's when the floor under him heaved. His wife screamed, and the bird fell out of her hands.

"Take Ranger and get to the basement," the man yelled as he flung open the back door. "You'll be safe there. Run, for God's sake. Run."

He hit the ground and sank into ankle-deep mud. Before he could catch his breath, his house slid past him, tumbling down the mountain, followed by a crest of silt that caught him in its wake. He surfed, riding a breaker of muck, while his house disintegrated before his eyes.

* * *

It had been five days since the mud slides. Beth had been paged Tuesday, but this was one time she couldn't respond immediately; AT&T had assigned her to the State Department and she'd only been on the job two days. Other search teams had been called in, but by Friday afternoon the woman was still missing and VDES called again. Beth would join them at around 0800 hours, she said. And she would be bringing an operational member of her own group, Search Services America, as backup.

Beth was not prepared for the devastation that met her. The distant hills and meadows were lush green, thick with forest and early spring grass. Here the valley, in stark contrast, more resembled a moonscape transported to earth. Whole hillsides had slid away like so much icing off a cake, depositing a scree of rocks and stones in their wake. The fledgling stems of future golden corn lay smothered under a wide swath of red Virginia clay. A herd of Black Angus poked their cow snouts around uprooted trees and plopped belly-deep into the thick sludge with a loud mooing when they lost their footing.

The deputy who'd been assigned to guide them pointed up a mountainside smeared with long, dark gashes. "That's where the house used to be." And Beth could see where the brick home had taken its long, unwanted ride into the valley.

She took note that the old stream had forced a tributary through a clutch of boulders up and off to her left and pointed it out to the volunteer firefighter she'd brought with her. "Blair, you and Duchess take the eastern bank of the old stream; I'll go up the middle between that and the new one." She pointed to a tangle of fallen trees a half mile ahead. "That's our meeting point. We'll keep in touch by radio."

The young man nodded understanding. "Find 'em," he ordered the small black and tan shepherd waiting eagerly by his side. Together, dog and master plunged into the field of mire in the direction Beth had decreed.

The skies had cleared, but teased the humans off and on with a dark face. Beth noticed a slight, blond woman standing off to one side, hands thrust into a denim jacket. She seemed to fold into herself as if wanting to disappear. "Who's that?"

The sheriff turned away so the girl couldn't read his lips. "That's the daughter. She's been hanging around since we started."

"It's her mother we're looking for," Beth murmured and took off to her own designated search area.

They hadn't made it halfway across the field when Czar honed in on a particular rock. To Beth's surprise her dog's pink tongue attacked the mound, licking its muddy surface as if it were a haunch of beef. She stubbed the rock with her toe. It *was* a haunch of beef. Czar's expression spoke volumes. *Glory Hallelujah! Yes!*

"No, Czar. You don't need that," Beth admonished.

Czar's head drooped; then he bounded another few feet, parked himself beside a mound of dirt, and immediately began to dig. Another heap of rotting meat was revealed. "Sorry." Beth smiled. "Different *napu.*"

The shepherd found other "rocks" as he and his mistress worked their way up the streams. Beth figured the unfortunate couple must have had at least two giant freezers in their home. After a few more chidings, Czar realized the wonderful treats were not for him this day.

The shepherd sniffed and burrowed on farther, but he gave Beth no alerts. They swept five acres, seven. Czar was suddenly interested in two huge boulders that had married in the muck. He lifted a mud-heavy paw and worried the opening between them, then disappeared. Beth hadn't realized how deep the void retreated. Ten seconds later, a head and ears peeked back up. This was not an alert. "Well, what?"

Czar disappeared again, and once more his head popped out of the gloom of the rocks. Now Beth could see from the way his back was arching that Czar was pawing at something. She climbed into the darkness to join him—nothing. Czar scrabbled hard beneath a rock, but there was nothing there either. Beth couldn't imagine what he was doing. "Show me."

Czar thrust his muzzle down hard, gave a little tug, and slowly pulled something toward her. It was a socked foot. Beth had looked straight at the victim and hadn't seen a thing. "Let's go. It's okay. Good dog. Good dog." She glanced at her watch. After five days of fruitless searching by others, it had taken the shepherd a mere fifty-five minutes to find the missing woman.

Beth climbed into the open field and turned on her radio. "Blair, Blair, come in, we have a find, status three." Before Blair could reply, a voice interrupted the transmission.

"Did I hear a status three?" Base radio had picked up.

"Confirmed," Beth said. In the parlance of search and rescue she had just told command camp that the victim was dead.

She felt tired all of a sudden, and dirty. She hooked the radio back onto her belt and ruffled Czar's fur. "A good bath tonight, my friend," she murmured. "For both of us."

An odd feeling that she was being watched made Beth turn. Not twenty yards away, the slender daughter followed her every move. She must have slogged her way through the mud and sneaked up when Beth and Czar were finding her mother.

The girl's presence bothered Beth. She didn't want to react to a stranger's naked grief. Yet when the medics and sheriff arrived, Beth took Czar and tacked a path across the field toward her.

The daughter couldn't wait. She stumbled forward to meet them and fell on Beth, sobbing. Beth wrapped her arms around sharp-boned shoulders and rocked the daughter's thin form close.

"Thank you. Thank you. You found my mother, didn't you?" the girl gasped when she finally caught her breath.

"Czar found her."

The young woman pulled away and stared at the dog whose white body was streaked with the red clay of Virginia. "Thank you, Czar," she whispered, then turned to Beth. "You love your dog, don't you?"

The question startled. "He's my partner, my best friend. Yes."

"Our dog's name was Ranger. My mother adored her. I found her smashed against a rock the first day, but they won't let me go back to get her." The girl's eyes were enormous with grief. "Ranger was my mother's baby. If I could bring her out and bury her . . ." She couldn't finish.

Beth hugged the girl one more time. "Let me see what I can do."

The sheriff looked distracted when she made the request, but Beth wasn't fazed. "Look, it means a lot to the daughter right now. She's shattered. Would it be so difficult to bring the dog out? If it were Czar, it'd be the least I'd expect."

"It's not something we usually do, but this situation is unusual." The sheriff bullhorned his hands around his mouth. "Bring an extra body bag over here. Follow that woman." He nodded toward the frail blonde. "Okay, missy, we'll get your dog for you."

The daughter clasped Beth's hands between her own, fighting the tears. "I'll never forget. Never."

Not knowing—the truth, the location, the reason, the denouement—is one of the most frustrating experiences of even our daily lives. Not knowing what has happened to a loved one—not being able to provide a decent burial, not being allowed to acknowledge closure to the end of a life—is a kind of torture. The pain and sorrow of it can scar a soul forever.

Once again, Beth Barkley was shown the true meaning of closure. As for Czar, he'd scented death one more time. Soon he would be surrounded by it.

CHAPTER 20

DISASTER—
OKLAHOMA CITY

AFTERMATH

In the morning
Between the screams
Under the dust
Amidst the scared people
Around the broken glass
Out in the air
Beyond the fallen walls
With the hurt babies
Above the sad earth
On the people's minds
Is DISASTER

SHANNA DEAKINS, 13
Deer Creek Middle School,
Oklahoma City

April 24, 1995, Second Shift

Czar was confused. He was alerting every two seconds—on every trickle of blood, every shred of skin he came across. Beth understood it would take a few minutes for her partner to acclimatize himself tonight. The blast that had blown the center out of the Alfred P. Murrah Federal Building had been so ferocious it had vaporized flesh. But her dog had to be reminded, and quickly, that it was bodies he needed to indicate in the saturation of death about them.

"That's good," Beth praised as his black nose sniffed a tangle of human viscera that had wrapped around a piece of rebar. Czar's eyes locked on his mistress. This was not the fulsome enthusiasm he was used to when he made a find. He placed a stiff paw tentatively on another bloodied piece of intestine, and Beth winced. "Good," she encouraged mildly, and moved him forward without another word.

It was eerie, Beth thought, how the sights and sounds of this disaster were like no other in her experience. There was none of the jumble of wreckage and twisted corners so familiar after the destruction wrought by a hurricane or earthquake. Instead, it was as if each floor of the federal building had exhaled upward, then come down together with the same precise angulation, spilling its chaos from within.

Unlike the puny illuminations cobbled together in other emergencies, the monstrous floodlights that played their harsh, white glare upon this building left nothing hidden. Beth preferred not to read the neat little desk plaques spelling names and titles. She didn't want to wonder about the chewed rim of a paper cup stained with morning coffee, about an office cluttered with memos and family photos, a desk still standing, pristine and tidy as a priest's altar. How little it all mattered now.

The noise was muted on the seventh floor. Beth knew they were on Level Seven, because it had green carpet. It was the same industrial green covering she'd seen from the street, dangling like sodden ribbon over a concrete precipice. Down below, the crashing and banging of huge dump trucks unloading debris, the shrill piercing of whistles, the shouted instructions of team leaders were an assault on the senses of both human and animal.

She watched Czar wedge his front shoulders between two blocks that had collided in the blast and formed a low tunnel. He backed out slowly, bent his foreleg, and dropped it heavily. This was different from his previous erratic signals. Beth didn't respond; she wanted the surety of her dog's alert.

Czar lifted his paw once again in a grave repeat. Beth squatted beside him and squinted into the tunnel. "Oh good boy, good Czar," she praised with all the fervor of old. Her dog had gotten it right. She turned to the two extrication specialists who copied her steps. "You'll be able to bring a body out here."

Dawn was brightening the sky when Beth led Czar off the rubble pile for a break. Garrett Dyer, the search manager for Task Force #1 from Virginia, had decreed that they rotate every thirty minutes. The firefighter understood the toll on both dogs and people. He knew his team had hoped desperately to find survivors, but five days after the blast they had recognized that all there was left to do was body recovery.

As the night wore down, Beth felt extraordinarily pleased to see Garrett's strong brown face and hear his contained authority order, "Your turn. Take twenty."

Twenty minutes. It was understood that twenty minutes was all they should take to rest their dogs. Two huge

FEMA tents were set up in the parking lot across from the federal building for that specific purpose.

Czar was drawn to the second tent. He'd claimed his favorite spot earlier in the night and now snuggled his tired self into its soft cloud of blanket. Beth eased off her helmet and goggles, dropped her pack, and flopped down beside him.

For the umpteenth time this shift she blessed the person or persons unknown who had layered the far corner of the tent three-deep with blankets. Whoever it was had guessed that the animals and their handlers would crawl down from the rubble of the Murrah building, sticky and sweaty, but minutes later be shaking with cold from the chilling rain. They'd set a big heater in the middle to churn out warmth against the thirty-five-degree night.

The throw on which Czar lay was truly beautiful—cozy, enveloping as a mother's embrace. Beth let her hands play in thick wool until her fingertips identified its luxury—llama hair. It was hard to appreciate the design because the blanket's deep cinnamon browns were smeared with the mud and diesel oil tracked in by dogs and boots from the outside. She wondered who'd donated this gorgeous covering. They must have known it couldn't be protected. That filth and grime must, by the very nature of the job, be ground into its precious weft and warp.

She propped her head on Czar's belly and fought the desire to surrender to the beguiling softness of the llama-hair blanket. Twenty minutes was hardly long enough in this safe place. Beth gazed up at the plastic-coated ceiling above her and reflected upon the evil that had been done to the citizens of Oklahoma City and the out-pouring of goodness in its wake.

Her thoughts drifted to the local veterinarians. "We will always be here. Twenty-four hours a day. No dogs will get hurt on this mission without our being there to take care of them."

Her fingers traced a grease spot by her hip. She remembered the fear in El Salvador, the paranoia in Armenia. Beth smiled in the dim light. How different was the attitude of the people of this city.

An anger was taking hold, a cold determination. The citizens of Oklahoma City deserved the best she had to give. The resolve infused her with new energy. She stood and stretched, fitted on her helmet, and tucked in her short, blond hair. Czar scrambled up, ready to work, as always. She took his face between her hands, and dropped a kiss on the great head of her best friend. "Let's go to it."

Their twelve-hour shift was over. Beth's first order of business when she came off the "pile," as the team called the federal building, was to decontaminate herself and Czar. It was a weary process after a night of searching. First a thorough scrubdown of her own body; then an hour of splashing her dog through the equivalent of sheep dip in the decontamination tent next to the Murrah building's parking garage; followed by a trudge to the bathrooms of the adjoining courthouse building to rinse and dry him; a bus trip to the Myriad Center; then, before she could eat or sleep, Czar had to have play time.

It was a necessary and mandatory process. The rescue workers and their dogs were constantly exposed to body fluids that could infect them with hepatitis, AIDS, or any number of communicable diseases.

At last it was done.

A weary Beth Barkley trudged up the ramp into the

loading dock of the Myriad Center, the home away from home for the nearly four hundred rescue workers FEMA had summoned from around the nation. It was a cavernous space, crammed with tables piled high with clothing, bedding, personal supplies, anything anybody could need. A waft of freshly baked apple turnovers tickled her nose and her tummy growled.

"You need anything this morning?" A plump, pleasant-faced woman opened her arms over the array of sundries displayed on the table before her. "Perfume? A little spritz of 'Charlie'? Take that smell away."

Beth smiled. "No thanks. But I did forget my toothpaste."

"Great. We got Colgate, Crest, Aquafresh—you want your teeth whiter, we got Rembrandt."

"Crest will do fine."

Czar's mind was on other things. The dog had already secured her place in line at the buffet. Beth picked up a tray and studied the plethora of steel steam tables. She pronounced a silent blessing upon the Oklahoma Restaurant Association, and the volunteers who cooked and served the rescue workers.

It was 10:30 A.M.—dinnertime for the partners. Beth passed by the scrambled eggs and bacon and headed for the roast beef. First order—Czar's favorite—green beans, lots of them.

She slid her loaded tray on a table next to Heidi Yamaguchi. Fuyu, Heidi's new dog, snored contentedly, her slim muzzle resting on her empty plate. Jean and Regina, who rounded out the dog team of Task Force #1 from Fairfax, had already gone to the women's sleeping quarters. Conversation was nonexistent. Both women were too tired to talk. Their exchange of nods said it all.

After dinner, dog and mistress could sleep. Beth walked to her cot, unzipping her coveralls. She paused and smiled. Neatly folded on top of the bed was yesterday's search uniform, smelling of Tide, all stains carefully removed. Even her team insignias had been ironed with care.

On the pillow were two Fanny Farmer mints, two Milkbones, and a handwritten note.

Dear Rescue Worker,

I again thank you for your extraordinary help. In our eyes you are heroes. I am sure it is destroying to see some of the things you see, but some way God will see you through it. I think it is extra heroic that you risk your life to save another. I hope that when you go home you value your love for your family and friends.

> In Christ's name,
> Ashley Banister, 12, Oklahoma City

Beth folded the note against her heart as she slept that night.

AGAPÉ

The botanical gardens across the street from Oklahoma City's convention center was the place of choice to de-stress the dogs every morning. Even though this April had been colder and wetter than usual, the grounds were green with new grass. Young shoots garlanded the trees, announcing the end of their winter hibernation. The walkways were redolent with masses of lilac and apple blossom—a welcome distraction from the dirt, choking dust, and concrete.

The gardens became a gathering place for rest and recreation for all the FEMA teams. For Beth it was like old-home week. Today she spotted a handsome young firefighter from Metro-Dade. "Skip Fernandez! How's your beautiful Aspen doing?"

"She's fine, how's our terrible Czar? I haven't seen you."

"You got the day shift. We come on at night."

The two friends watched Czar and Skip's golden retriever exchange territory markings on the roots of an oak.

"Bruce, Hunter's looking real good," she called to the handler from Seattle. "You know Skip and Aspen, don't you?"

Bruce wrung Skip's hand. "I saw your golden working yesterday. Nice dog."

The botanical gardens were the one retreat for the canine handlers and their animals. It didn't take long for the citizens of the city to discover this refuge. As each day passed, more and more came to say thank you.

The four dogs from Task Force #1, Beth and Heidi's white German shepherds and Jean and Regina's black Labradors, drew men, women, and children like magnets. "Our dogs look like a couple of matched pairs," Beth joked as she freed Czar from his leash.

A couple with a small, blond child in tow watched the dogs with indulgent smiles. The father strode up to Beth and her colleagues. "My wife and I just want to shake your hands," he said. "How can we ever thank you for coming?"

The four women chatted for a few minutes—all inter-action with the Oklahomans was special and welcome—

and drifted their separate ways to let their dogs explore. And that would have been the end of this exchange, too, except that Czar took it into his head to stop tumbling Heidi's Fuyu, and lope back to his mistress.

The blond child let go of her mother's hand and pointed. "Hero dog," she said and waddled toward the white shepherd.

Oh, no. This was Czar's play time. He was like Winnie-the-Pooh's Tigger—"jouncy, flouncy, bouncy, pouncy . . . full of fun, fun, fun," and the toddler was directly in his path.

Beth ran to intervene—too late. Czar bounded toward the little girl, lowered his head, and butted her joyously from behind. The child sprawled face first on the wet grass and promptly bawled.

Beth got to her first. "She's all right," she called to the mother, whose face had whitened to match Czar's fur. "Down," she commanded her animal as she lifted the little girl to her feet. From the tone of her voice Czar knew he'd done wrong. He dropped on his haunches, and hung his head. But Beth could see his eyes watching like those of an inquisitive magpie.

The father wiped his hands on the pants of his jeans while his wife held her daughter's head against her skirt. "Shush now," she said.

"I'm so sorry," Beth apologized, then squatted beside the child. "My dog means no harm. It's just that you're the same height as he is and he wanted to play."

The girl peeked from behind the protection of her mom's leg. "Hero dog?" she questioned. The mother smiled. The father took Beth's hand in his. "We meant what we said. We don't know how to express our gratitude. We know your dog was just letting off steam. Think nothing of it. God bless you."

The week went on. The arduous work of search, broken by long downtimes exiled from the "pile," took its toll. The rescue workers could not be exposed to the car-sized chunks of concrete—"widowmakers"—that dangled by wires, thin iron rods, copper pipes, ready to drop. The lesson was learned the hard way. The nurse who'd been crushed as she rushed to help would never be forgotten. The widowmakers had to be harnessed and winched to the ground as excavation progressed.

On this particular night, Beth noticed Czar stiffen, as if in shock, when he alerted. As she signaled yet another body to the heavy rescue men, he lay down and stared straight ahead for a minute before going on.

Once again Czar was showing more clearly than words his feelings about the wash of death that emanated from every void of the building. Beth thought about those who ridiculed the idea that dogs were pack animals, and that people were their pack. She'd never understand that point of view. If nothing else, they reflected their handlers' stress.

It was a subdued and exhausted dog and mistress that trudged into the Myriad Center the next morning. Beth fed and watered Czar, but had little appetite herself. All she wanted was some sleep.

But the good citizens of Oklahoma had another surprise in store for the rescue workers. A line of tables draped with white cotton sheets, surrounded by moveable partitions for privacy, waited down the hall from their sleeping quarters. Next to each was a shining-faced masseuse. Attached to the pockets of their uniforms were pinned name tags. "Myotherapists Association Disaster Support Team."

"Oh, yes," Beth breathed, dropped onto the nearest trestle, and gave herself up to skillful fingers. She was about to enter dreamland when a girlish voice penetrated her consciousness.

"Your dog has such a presence."

Nobody had ever described Czar that way before. Irascible, yes. Impossible, certainly. But presence? Beth opened her eyes to see a girl with the ripped body of an athlete petting the shepherd who'd stretched out next to her table. "Thank you."

"I know how to massage an animal," the young woman continued. "You start with their feet. . . ." She lifted Czar's back paw and kneaded his pad. Czar pulled his leg away and sat.

"Try his back," Beth suggested. It was exactly what the masseuse had just finished doing on her, and it felt divine.

The girl squatted and worked her fingers down Czar's spine, feeling the knots, working them. Czar swayed to some inner symphony. He drifted so far left Beth was sure he'd fall on his keister. The "dog masseuse" smiled and eased the unprotesting animal to the floor. He relaxed his head on his front paws and snored. "I'll massage all his muscles; they need it as much as we do. My name is Sylvia, by the way."

Whatever you say, Sylvia.

From then on, Sylvia was at the Myriad Center every morning at ten. Czar would run up and place his paws on her chest and yatter his happiness to see her. Sylvia's massages got longer and longer. She took to bringing dog cookies and toys as part of her therapy. The treatments mellowed Czar to the point that Beth couldn't believe his behavior.

AT&T and Southwestern Bell had set up telephones for the rescue workers in the eating area. They could call anyone, anywhere, anytime—free. One noontime, Beth sat with her back against the wall, catching up on news and messages with Gayle Arrington.

"Is Siri behaving himself?"

"As always, Beth. He's such a love."

"And little Too?"

"You'd never know that dog had heart trouble the way she plays with Siri all day."

Beth smiled. Five years ago she'd brought the white ball of fluff who was not expected to live more than a few months to a dear friend with the same diagnosis. And here they were, stronger than ever, visiting nursing homes and children's hospitals. She was so caught up in memories of Gayle and Too that she didn't see what mischief Czar was up to.

The shepherd sprawled not three feet away. Beth had gotten an extra portion of green beans and thought Czar was feasting in uninterrupted peace. But she noticed that as people walked by, they started to giggle. She turned to see what was so funny.

Czar had straightened his big mass smack on his haunches and was eyeing a toddler whose dark curls were inches from his fangs. She hadn't quite broken the dog of the habit of "eating kids." The child held Czar's dinner plate. How had he gotten it away from the dog? "Catch you later, Gayle."

"Thank you for coming," the lad said gravely to Czar as he picked up a skinny green bean, and dangled the vegetable in front of the dog's muzzle. Beth scooted toward the boy and the shepherd, but Czar was quicker. He stretched his jaws within the child's reach and opened wide. With a gleeful gurgle, the toddler dropped the bean precisely and accurately into the waiting mouth. Czar swallowed and opened his muzzle again.

"Thank you for coming," the child repeated and dropped another green bean into waiting jaws. Beth didn't believe what she was witnessing. Czar did not snap, growl, or take the toddler's finger off. He sat before the boy—a perfect angel, ears up, attentive. Beth could swear he was smiling.

She sidled over, just to be on the safe side. "My dog's name is Czar, and green beans are his favorite."

"I know," the child replied. "He told me."

"Oh, he did, did he?" Beth said, and made a mental note to see that Czar got massages for the rest of his life.

Night after night Beth was drawn to the refuge of the tent with the beautiful llama blanket. Night after night she and Czar sank into its thick, heavy warmth. She would never know what made her turn up a corner one 3 A.M. A plastic bag, pinned to the underside, protected a sheet of yellow legal paper folded in half. Beth unpinned the plastic and spread out the paper. Four simple sentences stared up at her. The realization of what they meant took a few seconds to sink in.

The throw on which Beth lay had been brought back from South America by Patty Herson's late brother. His last request before he died was that it be given to his daughter when she turned twenty-one. But Patty Herson felt that the rescue workers might need it more these nights than her family did. All she asked was that, if it were possible, the throw be returned.

Beth stared at the oil, grime, dirt, and dog hair that desecrated the beautiful object. She thought of all the kindness, generosity, unselfish acts, and sacrifices of the people of Oklahoma City. A long-forgotten word crept back into memory.

Agapé—in college, Beth had studied the ancient Greek word. A kind of love that is not sexual or emotional but a deep, caring gratitude and appreciation that overlooks all faults and flaws. Beth had volunteered over seventeen years in search and rescue, yet she'd never quite experienced it before. Awe, yes—in Armenia and Salvador. But never anything like this outpouring of love from the men, women, and children of Oklahoma City.

Beth vowed Patty Herson would get her treasure back. She'd take advantage of the UPS offer to mail for free, and ship the blanket to herself in Virginia. She would wash and purify the lovely thing, and slip a note of her own in the package before posting it back:

I just wanted you to know, the first two nights this blanket kept firefighters warm, and after that a grateful rescue dog and his person.

Beth Barkley
Task Force # 1, Fairfax, Virginia

Beth's fingers lifted from the blanket to trace the outline of the American flag on the embroidered patch over her right breast. Their tips slid over the FEMA emblem on the sleeve of her navy sweatshirt. They drifted to explore the Fairfax County Fire Department insignia on the left arm. Finally, they came to rest on the Velcro name tag that told her name and position of canine handler.

And she felt proud.

GOOD-BYE

"Tonight's our last shift." The word flew from one to the other of the men and women of the Virginia contingent. Task Force #1 had been expecting it. As in all disasters, there is a point of diminishing return; after seven days the six teams of rescue workers called by FEMA from all over the country had worked the pile from top to bottom. They'd brought out 169 dead.

Beth thought she was prepared for the inevitable letdown that comes after enormous emotion and energy is expended. But try as she might she could muster no excitement for going home this last Saturday afternoon. A nagging feeling of something left undone was draining the last of her stamina as surely as if she were being sucked down a sinkhole.

The knowledge of their leaving seemed to affect the other members of the team the same way. They wandered aimlessly about the Myriad Center, feet dragging, barely a smile between them.

Beth couldn't remember how they all gathered together. She just knew they were all there. The firefighters, doctors, heavy rescue personnel, paramedics, technical support, dog handlers, all sixty-two members of Task Force #1 bunched in little knots like they were waiting for the priest to deliver the last rites.

"We can't just leave."

"We hung our flag on Murrah."

"Everybody else's flags are up there too."

"We could paint 'Our team was here.' " Whistles of protest met this suggestion.

"We don't mean something for *us*. We should do something for the people." The statement was flat, strong; a murmur of consent passed among them. All knew, as if connected by a psychic cord, that the man who spoke had not referred to the living souls of Oklahoma City, although they had carved their names into each of the task force members' hearts. He meant the victims.

A male voice broke the buzz of discussion. "How about we forget the buses tomorrow morning?"

"What d'you mean?"

"How about we walk? We send our gear back on the transport and all of us walk back . . . but do it in silence. A silent tribute."

Nobody said anything. Then very quietly Beth heard, "Not bad. I'll go for it."

"How do we do it?"

"In formation. Professional."

"I like it."

Another silence.

"It's settled then."

There was a collective sigh of assent.

Beth checked her watch. It had taken less than fifteen minutes for all sixty-two people of varying backgrounds, personalities, and points of view to come to agreement. Tomorrow Task Force # 1 from Virginia would walk as one, as men and women who had finished their mission but needed to offer a tribute. The March of Silence would be their legacy.

* * *

The garage that was the staging area for all operations was just like any other: "I" beam supports, bare concrete floors, open to the outside from the waist up. Yet this base camp had been their second home the last week. Beth made her way to the corner where the local veterinarians manned their posts.

"Czar and I want to say good-bye," she said to the slightly balding doctor with the crinkles around his eyes.

"We'll miss you. Come back and see us at a better time."

"Thank you for the hair dryers."

A big grin deepened the lines that radiated good humor. He knew exactly what Beth was referring to. One of the first items the vets had given the handlers was huge professional dryers like the ones once seen in grooming salons. It had cut the drying time for the dogs after their decontamination bath from hours to minutes.

"I can't let Czar go without a last treat," the doctor said.

Beth followed his eyes over neatly stacked blankets, kennels, bags of treats, heaps of toys. "I think he'll like this." He held out a giant squeak toy.

Beth smiled. "That'll do very nicely. Say good-bye to everyone for us."

Her next stop was across the far wall of the garage, where Metro-Dade had staked their territory. It was the first time Beth had worked with the Miami crew since dogs had joined their ranks. The four-legged Florida recruits were not used to the wet cold that seemed to creep into the very marrow of one's bones. Their handlers had taken blankets from the vets, laid them on the concrete, and commandeered lights on metal tripods, adjusting to three feet—dog's height. No animal of theirs was going to suffer. Skip Fernandez, the search-dog leader, made sure the canines of Metro-Dade bathed in well-deserved warmth between shifts.

"Good-bye," she said to the men she'd gotten to know over the years. "See you around."

"See you, Beth," they said in turn. Some accompanied their farewells with hugs, some with handshakes.

A renewed sense of purpose took Task Force #1 from Fairfax, Virginia, through the last hours. The morning came quickly. Their job here was done, and Garrett's calm voice was giving one last order. "Time to go, guys. Dogs in front."

In squadron formation, the sixty-two men, women, and dogs who had answered the summons to emergency from Oklahoma City marched out to the street for their last special good-bye.

The March of Silence was not the end for Beth and Czar. Four days after she'd shipped the cinnamon llama blanket back to Patty Herson, the Oklahoma City woman called. She was delirious with delight. She'd never expected to see the treasure again. "And that would have been all right with me and my niece," she hastened to assure. "But this is so much better."

Out of the tragedy that changed the way a nation looked at itself came a wonderful friendship. Patty Herson represented for Beth all the Oklahomans whose hands stretched out to her in grateful friendship; whose words soothed her pain while their own was still apparent deep in their eyes; whose kindness and generosity she could never forget.

The spirit of the people of that city, of that state, had managed through sheer goodness to turn a monster's attempted triumph into dross.

AFTERWORD

Beth's love of her volunteer work has never flagged. A new dog, Jadzia, is in training in the household.

Every month someone goes missing. Every month the team responds.

In the fall of 1996, she and Czar responded to the devastation of the barrier islands in the wake of Hurricane Fran.

In the United States, domestic terrorism is a new emergency that sadly will not go away. Beth and Czar were one of the teams on call for immediate dispatch to Atlanta during the Olympic Games if it became necessary.

It will not be the last time.

For Beth Barkley, Czar "the Terrible," and those to follow, the journey continues.

BETH BARKLEY

Beth Barkley, a former classical vocalist, has had seventeen years' experience in the discipline of search and rescue. She is a state resource for the Virginia Department of Emergency Services, and a canine search specialist for the Fairfax County FEMA Disaster Response Team. She was a ten-year volunteer with DOGS East, Inc., where she had served as training director. She is the founder and training director of Search Services America, Inc., a nonprofit canine search group whose members are drawn from law enforcement and firefighting communities. Beth has been an instructor at the Ground Search and Rescue College of the VDES, the Federal Emergency Management Agency Canine Disaster Schools, and Managing the Search Function and Field Team Member courses. She has responded to international calls at the request of the Office of Foreign Disaster Assistance.

She is trainer and partner of Panda, Sirius, SAR Czar, and Jadzia, and recently started her own search-and-rescue training school, Find 'Em K-9 SAR, in Falls Church, Virginia.

For those interested, a "SAR DOG DIRECTORY," listing search-dog groups around the country, can be obtained from:

THE NATIONAL ASSOCIATION FOR SEARCH AND RESCUE
4500 SOUTHGATE PLACE
SUITE 100
CHANTILLY, VIRGINIA 20151

DIAL 911

by Joan E. Lloyd & Edwin B. Herman

Imagine your worst fear. A loved one falls to the floor,
unconscious. A car hurtles out of control at fifty miles
per hour. An infant ingests poison. You dial 911, and
the emergency medical technicians answer the call.
Now here are their stories, based on
the authors' own experiences as members of
a volunteer ambulance corps.

From the most traumatic cases to the most bizarre,
every call is recounted in exact detail—and with
absolute authenticity. DIAL 911 takes you inside the
world of emergency medicine in a way you've never
seen before.

Published by Ivy Books.
Available in bookstores everywhere.

LIFE AND DEATH...

The people in these books face both on a daily basis.
Here's your opportunity to walk in their shoes.